·COMMON· PLANTS ·AS· ·NATURAL· REMEDIES

What right have you, O passer-by-the-way
to call any flower a weed?
Do you know its merits, its virtues,
its healing qualities?
Because a thing is common
shall you despise it?

·COMMON· PLANTS ·AS· ·NATURAL· REMEDIES

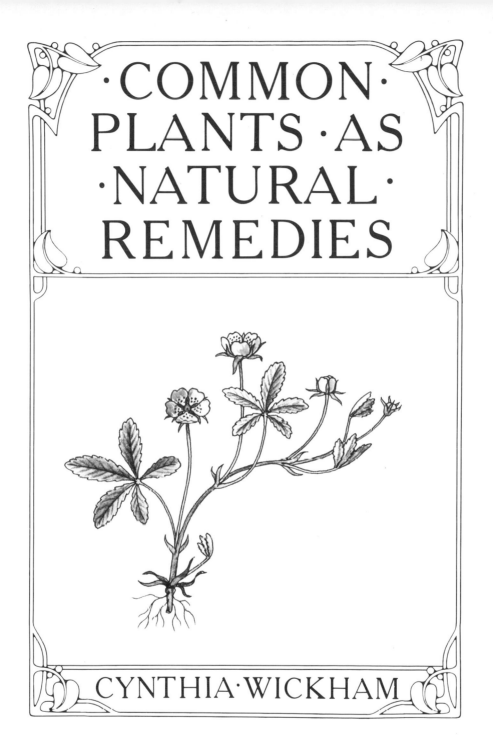

CYNTHIA·WICKHAM

FREDERICK MULLER LIMITED · LONDON

Contents

First published in Great Britain 1981 by
Frederick Muller Limited, London, SW19 7JU
Reprinted 1982

Text copyright © 1981 Cynthia Wickham
Illustrations copyright © Ringier & Co AG, Zofingen

British Library Cataloguing in Publication Data

Wickham, Cynthia · Common plants as natural remedies · 1. Herbs –
Therapeutic use · 1. Title · 615′ .321   RS164 ·
ISBN 0-584-10475-8
ISBN 0-584-11030-8 pbk

The 15 teas starting with Headache Tea on p. 137 and the Other Concoctions
on p. 140 were suggested by the Swiss homeopath, Dr Robert Quinche.
The foreword by E. F. Schumacher is reprinted by permission from *The
Virtuous Weed* by Joy Griffith-Jones, Blond & Briggs, 1977.
Thanks are due to William Collins & Co. Ltd. for permission to quote material
on p. 34 from *Health Secrets of Plants and Herbs* by Maurice Mességué.

Printed and bound in Great Britain by
Fakenham Press Limited, Fakenham, Norfolk

Where, What, How?

Which medicinal plants affect which organs of the body
The figures refer to the page numbers of the plant descriptions or the tea mixtures

Breathing passages
Sore throat 60, 100, 120
Inflammation of the throat 60, 78, 100
Coughing 16, 18, 28, 78, 116, 120, 139
Convulsive coughing 18, 80, 116
Colds, flu 32, 94, 96, 102, 140

Moving organs (limbs)
Blood effusions 26, 62
Rheumatism, gout 46, 92, 96, 104, 114, 130, 140

Heart, circulation
Stimulation of the heart 66, 136, 140
Stimulation of the circulation 62, 139
High blood pressure 22, 48, 136
Nervous heart trouble 48, 108
Venal stoppages 118
Varicose veins, haemorroides, 18, 44, 118

Urinal passages
Stimulating the kidneys 34, 46, 52, 86, 104, 132
Kidneys, bladder, 52, 68, 86, 126, 138

Nervous system
Nervous stimulation 66
Quieting the nerves, insommnia 24, 74, 76, 82, 106, 108, 122, 139
Pains 80
Migraines 24, 139
Inflammation of the eyes 64

Sexual organs
Monthly trouble 18, 58, 76, 82, 90, 140

Heavy regular bleeding 30, 44, 68
Menopausal trouble 58, 68
White discharge 30, 58
Prostate trouble 86

Metabolism
Purification of the blood 20, 22, 34, 36, 46, 50
Anaemia 46
Reducing a fever 32, 94, 96, 102, 114
Inducing sweating 56, 92, 102
Stimulating the metabolism 66
Diabetes 124

Skin
Skin rash, acne, eczema 36, 38, 42, 50, 52, 100, 138
Boils 38, 60, 92
Wounds 44, 60, 64, 70, 76, 86, 100
Burns 16, 44
Warts 54

Digestive tract
Weak stomach 32, 66, 72, 78, 84, 88, 98, 100, 110, 132, 140
Colic, stomach cramps 18, 84, 90
Flatulence 74, 98
Intestinal catarrh 28, 64, 76, 112
Diarrhoea 30, 44, 124, 140
Constipation 40, 90, 92, 140
Liver-bile stimulation 20, 36, 54, 70, 74, 76, 88, 128, 140

Foreword

The more we learn about nature the more we must doubt our theories. Evolution, for instance, claims that what exists today is through natural selection, that nature is a utilitarian system allowing survival only to the fittest as if designed by the engineers of a multi-national corporation. This view obscures the marvels of nature which is an artistic wonder, infinitely playful, subtle and inventive, whose wisdom we should be humbly eager to understand.

Alas, we approach nature in a very different spirit, as a system that requires continuous correction. How incompetent she is, allowing pests and diseases, iron to rust, useful substances to decay, and low parasites to flourish at the expense of higher creatures. All this has to be battled with. Cosmic incompetence has produced friends and enemies for us and once we know who is who, we know what to do—kill the enemy.

Among the enemies are weeds, useless and troublesome plants in cultivated land, springing up where not wanted. The multi-national corporation called nature has failed to develop effective weed-killers, but our own multi-nationals have succeeded where nature has failed. We can exterminate the weeds . . .

But do we really know what we are doing? Is this a matter for killing, or thoughtful, gentle, loving management? Is there really no virtue in weeds? Are they really unmanageable, so that there is no alternative to *herbicide?*

Let us study them, as our ancestors have done with science *and* sensitivity, and learn from nature. We can start, where we may expect the least, but can find enough for a lifetime, in our own backyard.

E. F. SCHUMACHER

The revival of interest in wild herbs and homeopathy

'Anything green that grew out of the mould
Was an excellent herb to our fathers of old.'

KIPLING

Many wild plants contain nutritional or healing properties once well known and now in the process of being rediscovered. What our 'fathers of old' knew by instinct, tradition and inherited knowledge is now proved scientifically by chemists in laboratories.

Most of these plants are known as 'weeds' because they are successful and strong, and mainly because they have a tendency to grow in the wrong place. After all a weed is only a plant growing where it is not wanted and usually very healthily and vigourously, and all those dandelions, nettles, plantains and yarrows were once highly prized because of their health-giving properties. One of the best and easiest ways to benefit from the properties of these plants is to use them for an infusion or tisane—lime flowers, mint, thyme, and camomile are only a few which are used in this way. A number of the herbs in this book, although growing wild in some parts of the world, as indeed all herbs were wild once, have to be cultivated in gardens in Britain and need a little cosseting and attention. Rosemary, bergamot and caraway, for instance, fall into this category.

It must be stressed that this is an account of various wild plants and their uses and properties, particularly with regard to herbal medicine and homeopathy. It is not a list of plants which may be picked and used by anybody, in fact some of them are dangerously toxic and clear warnings are given about these in the text. For those of them which are benign and safe to use recipes for infusions are given. It is not for a moment suggested that they are an alternative to conventional medicine for grave illnesses, but more that they might be considered mainly for their health-giving effect as a supplement to a diet or as tonics: plants to keep you well rather than plants to guarantee miraculous recoveries.

Many of the plants are well known as culinary herbs, such as thyme, sage and rosemary, and many as weeds we spend out time trying to erradicate from the garden, such as dandelion, plantain, elder and bramble.

It intensifies the pleasure of country walks when wild plants can be identified and recognised, and this book tells what a veritable medicine chest is found in every wood and hedgerow. Another thing to be stressed is that we have to be careful of wild plants, many of them are poisonous, and in some cases, particularly in the Umbellifer (parsley and carrot) family, the toxic ones are very hard to distinguish from the others. Something else to bear in mind is that there are other dangers from pollution, particularly from the chemicals used in crop spraying in the country, and no plants must be used which might be affected by these pollutants. Incidentally it is a sad fact that many so-called weeds are rich in nutritional elements for the soil itself, and the soil loses much of its richness without them. Many of these weeds are being wiped out by the use of pesticides. An American scientist, Luther Burbank, noticed that fields of wheat where flowers grew produced not only better flowers but better wheat. Experiments are going on now where birds are used to stop locust plagues, and ladybirds wage war on citrus pests, and these biological ways of control do nothing to upset the balance of nature as lethal chemicals do, and which end up killing off far more than the pests they were designed to eliminate.

There are many wild plants which are cultivated for the drug market, or gathered in controlled conditions, and are part of the stock of herbalists and homeopathic doctors. Generally speaking, it is better for the amateur to stick to the easily recognised plants, and certainly never to experiment with any which may have undesirable effects.

When picking herbs for drying or using fresh as tisanes it is best to use only those from your own garden, certainly only from places known to be free of pesticides. When it comes to the poisonous plants, such as henbane, bryony and mistletoe, it is advisable not to touch any of them but just to note and admire.

One of the earliest herbals, written over 5000 years ago in China sets out over a thousand remedies; the Egyptians used herbs in their surprisingly advanced medicine (an Egyptian doctor/herbalist explained the circulation of the blood in 3000 BC) and the ancient Babylonians and Assyrians did too. Hippocrates, the Greek 'father of medicine' wrote about treatment using the accumulated knowledge of thousands of years, and he also taught that the whole physical and psychological condition of the patient, not just one or two painful symptoms, must be taken into account.

All living creatures seem to have a remarkable capacity for self healing by natural methods; cats and dogs, for instance, eat grass when they need to make themselves sick. Herbal medicines became increasingly popular. The barbers amalgamated with the Royal College of Surgeons in 1540 and at this time, due to pressure from the barber-surgeons, Henry VIII instituted an Act of Parliament virtually persecuting herbalists and forbidding them to practice. The physicians and barbers, grew so powerful and so expensive, that poorer people could not afford treatment, so that finally, in 1542, herbalists were allowed to work again. One of the most famous of them was Nicholas Culpeper (1616–1654) whose *Compleat Herbal* has been in print ever since, and some of whose cures, though rather bewilderingly mixed up with astrology, are still in use today.

A system of natural healing found all over the world is known as the doctrine of signatures, and it works on the understanding that like cures like. At its most basic it means that plants with red flowers or leaf pattern are good for the blood, and those with heart shaped leaves are good for the heart. This idea led to such names as spleenwort, liverwort, heartsease and eyebright for plants. The like to like theory is at the basis of homeopathy, founded by Dr Samuel Hahnemann in Saxony (now part of East Germany). He said that if a drug produced results and symptoms similar to those of a disease then the use of it can help the body fight the disease. The other important point about homeopathy is that the individual's background, habits and general health are taken into account, and that any drugs given are specially mixed for one individual for his or her own particular needs and circumstances. In homeopathy some poisonous substances are used in miniscule quantities, as are other substances not derived from plants. This is where it differs from herbalism which uses only herbs, and non-toxic plants. Samuel Thompson made a reputation for his herbal remedies in America in the last century, and his type of herbalism was brought to this country by various practitioners.

There is now a branch of science called pharmacognosy which is devoted to testing and investigating the active principles of plants, and many of the ancient cures have been scientifically proved efficacious as the various elements in the plants are identified and analysed.

With the strong warnings and exceptions given above in mind, herbal remedies are relatively cheap for minor ailments. You can make them yourself at home, and can buy dried herbs and mixtures at a herbal supplier. Coughs and colds can be relieved by camomile, coltsfoot, comfrey and horsetail; elderflowers help toothache and are good for the skin; and eyebright and cornflowers are a tonic for the eyes. Insect bites and stings are soothed by the leaves of plantain and lemon balm, and for a general tonic infusions made from yarrow, nettle, sage and lemon balm are not only effective but delicious. The text describes the growing conditions of the plants in Great Britain, but many of them will grow successfully in very different conditions in other parts of the world. Almost all of them are also available in tincture or fluid extract form from herbalists.

Homeopathy may be defined as a system of medical practice founded by Hahnemann of Leipzig about 1796, according to which diseases are treated by the administration, usually in minute doses, of drugs which produce, in a healthy person, symptoms like those of the disease. The principle is described in the Latin adage—'similia similibus curantur' . . . or 'like cures like.'

9

At the age of 35 Hahnmann tried out on himself the drug quinine and developed a fever like that which quinine was used to cure. He experimented with other substances and came to the conclusion that like cures like, and believed that a drug acted by setting up an antagonistic fever which fought against the illness. In 1796 he named this new method of treatment 'homeopathy' from the two Greek words, 'homos' meaning 'like' and 'pathos' meaning 'suffering'. The remedies were simple animal, vegetable or mineral substances, all tried out on the healthy before being used on the sick. It was discovered that decreasing the amount given did not diminish the effectiveness, indeed the results seemed better when the amount of the drug was reduced almost to nothing. This discovery became known as the law of potencies and was a reason for the lack of belief in homeopathy, as people could not believe that such diluted, miniscule amounts of a drug could have any effect on a patient. In spite of this, and a great deal of hounding and scepticism, Hahnemann finally became internationally known, and homeopathy was well established in many countries at his death.

Hahnemann believed in treating the patient rather than the disease, and in speculating why people become ill he came to believe that illness is a way of expressing something by a patient, and that a doctor's job is to find the underlying cause as well as to remove the symptoms. In this he was in advance of his time, anticipating Freud's discoveries and even Freud's method of treatment, for homeopathic doctors encourage patients to talk about their life and circumstances, and it may well be that this interest encourages patients, putting them into a better state of mind and starting them on the way to curing themselves.

Some of the most important people associated with discoveries in medicine in general, and homeopathy in particular, are listed below.

DIOSCORIDES 1st century AD. Author of *De Materia Medica* in which the properties of over 500 plants are described. It was the leading work on pharmacalogy for over a thousand years and a basis for all the herbals of the Middle Ages.

GALEN 130–200 AD. A highly respected physician and an authority for over 1000 years, his work was still being studied in the 17th century.

HIPPOCRATES 460–*circa* 377 BC. The father of clinical medicine who established the scientific basis of therapeutic medicine.

PARACELSIUS 1490–1541. He sought new fields in medicine in the Renaissance and discovered the importance of precise dosage of chemical and natural substances.

PLINY THE ELDER 23–79 AD (died observing an erruption of Vesuvius). A Roman naturalist who wrote a *Natural History* in 37 volumes describing the beneficial plants used in his time.

THEOPHRASTUS 372–287 BC. A Greek philosopher, disciple of Plato and Aristotle, called the father of botany for his work on plants.

NICHOLAS CULPEPER 1616–1654. An astrologer-physician. After serving an apprenticeship to an apothecary he set up a practice in Spitalfields in 1640. He devoted much time to the study of astrology and medicine, fought on the Parliamentary side in the Civil War, and was wounded in the chest. His *Herbal* is still in print.

JOHN GERARD 1545–1611. An Elizabethan physician who was both a gardener and a philosopher, he published an *Anatomie of Plants* in 1597.

JOHN EVELYN 1620–1706. He is best known, like Pepys, for his Diaries, but in 1664 he published a book on practical arboriculture (tree growing) called *Sylva* which had a great influence, and he also published a number of translations from the French on architecture and gardening.

MAURICE MESSÉGUÉ is a herbalist and healer who lives in Provence in France. He is the son of a farm worker and much of his knowledge is traditional, having been handed down for generations. His reputation as a healer is worldwide and he has written several books on natural cures using plants, doing more than anybody to take these nature remedies out of the realm of the so-called 'cranks' and gaining a universal reputation for his successes.

Plants and their constituents

In ancient times many plants were valued because of their proven healing and soothing properties which were looked upon as magical, understandably, when leaves, flowers and fruits could cure or relieve illness. Scientists today can identify properties in plants which have these effects but in many ways this makes them no less magical or amazing. It has been estimated that one in seven of all plants has medicinal or curative powers, but only if carefully and properly chosen and carefully prepared.

ALKALOIDS Organic compounds containing nitrogen and affect the nervous system and blood vessels. They are toxic and correct dosage is vital. The first alkaloid to be chrystallised was morphine. The opium poppy produces about thirty alkaloids; nicotine is an alkaloid, similar to that in hemlock. Generally speaking they are bitter in taste. White bryony, greater celandine, henbane, butterbur, comfrey, mistletoe.

VITAMINS Are essential to good health and their deficiency produces diseases. Parsley, spinach, carrots, orange juice, flax, mallow.

ANTIBIOTICS Destroy or arrest the growth of micro-organisms. Moulds were used to cure infections in ancient Rome, and in the 12th century St Hildegard prescribed lichens and mosses to treat chills and fevers. Garlic contains an antibiotic.

HETEROSIDES Sugars or mucilages combined with active compounds which affect, selectively, various organs of the body. Most plants used in medicine contain either alkaloids or heterosides. Bearberry, meadowsweet, willow, shepherd's purse, hawthorn, horsetail, silver-weed, elder, masterwort, St John's wort, lady's mantle, tormentil, bramble, bilberry.

ESSENTIAL OILS AND RESINS Yarrow, camomile, arnica, marigold, cara-way, juniper, mint, restharrow, burnet saxifrage, rosemary, sage, thyme, lime.

BITTER COMPOUNDS Wormwood, arti-choke, yellow gentian, herb robert, hop, bog bean, dandelion.

SAPONOSIDES Increase the body's ability to absorb some active compounds such as calcium and silicon. Spinach, haricot beans, tomatoes, oats, horse chestnut, silver birch, cowslip, sanicle, soapwort, golden rod, mullein, heartsease.

ACIDS Raspberry, male fern.

MUCILAGES Plantain, mallow, coltsfoot.

INORGANIC COMPOUNDS Nettles.

The individual plants in the text

COLTSFOOT Contains mucilage; a soothing tonic and remedy for colds.

BUTTERBUR Contains an alkaloid, an

essential oil, tannin and mucilage; it is a heart stimulant, tonic, diuretic, a remedy for fevers and asthma.

DANDELION Bitter compounds and tannin; it is diuretic, tonic, a general stimulant.

GARLIC Antibiotic; it is a stimulant, and antiseptic, and cleanser.

COWSLIP Saponosides, a diuretic and sedative.

COMFREY Alkaloids, tannin, mucilages; used for coughs, throat, intestinal troubles, and as a dressing for wounds, fractures and sprains.

PLANTAIN Mucilage and heteroside; it is antidiarrhoeic, expectorant, emollient and vulnerary.

SILVERWEED Tannin, flavones; it is astringent and antispasmodic.

BOG BEAN A bitter compound; it is tonic and sedative.

SILVER BIRCH Saponosides; diuretic (leaves), stimulating bile (buds).

SOAPWORT The saponin content makes it purgative, diuretic and expectorant.

SANICLE Saponins; bitter, used to heal wounds, and as a gargle.

ALDER BUCKTHORN Contains glycosides; it is purgative, deruptive and diuretic.

HERB ROBERT Contains a bitter compound and tannins and an essential oil; it is astringent and sedative.

TORMENTIL Contains tannin, a glycoside and an acid; it is astringent.

STINGING NETTLE Acid, silicon, tannin, potassium and vitamins; it is haemostatic, antidiabetic and diuretic.

HAWTHORN Flavonoids; it is a strong tonic, antispasmodic and sedative.

HEARTSEASE Saponins, salicylates and a glycoside; it is diuretic, expectorant, deruptive and laxative.

HORSETAIL Rich in silica, glycosides, a saponiside and traces of alkaloids; it is diuretic, haemostatic, vulnerary, and a source of minerals.

GREATER CELANDINE Alkaloids with opium-like characteristics, essential oils and enzymes; it is toxic, narcotic, diuretic and purgative.

LIME Essential oil, glycosides, tannins, mucilage; lime is bechic, diaphoretic, antispasmodic and soothing.

LADY'S MANTLE Contains tannin, and is tonic, astringent and deruptive.

MALLOW Rich in mucilage, sugars, pectin, asperagine; it is emollient, and soothing.

ARNICA Essential Oil and heterosides; it is a stimulant for the circulation.

CAMOMILE Heterosides, an essential oil; it is carminative, soothing and antispasmodic.

ROSEMARY An essential oil; it is stimulant and antispasmodic; large quantities are toxic.

SHEPHERD'S PURSE Amino-alcohols, stops bleeding; it is hypertensive.

MARIGOLD An essential oil, a resin, saponin and a bitter compound; marigold is antiphlogistic, vulnerary and choleretic.

MASTERWORT An essential oil, heterosides; it is diuretic, diaphoretic and is a stomachic.

PEPPERMINT An essential oil, menthone, tannins and bitter compounds; it is aromatic, antispasmodic, carminative, tonic, stimulant, excitant and aphrodisiac.

ST JOHN'S WORT Essential oil, a glycoside; it is sedative, antidepressant, and antidiarrhoeic.

BURNET SAXIFRAGE Essential oil, tannin, and resin; it is antispasmodic, stomachic and diuretic.

HENBANE Poisonous. Contains alkaloids; it is sedative, analgesic and spasmolytic.

BERGAMOT Aromatic oil; sedative.

WORMWOOD Essential oil, a glycoside; wormwood is a bitter tonic, febrifuge, antiseptic, diuretic and a vermifuge.

GOLDEN ROD Saponins, an essential oil, bitter compound and tannin; it is diuretic, expectorant, anti-diarrhoeic.

CENTAURY Bitter compounds; choleretic, stomachic, and a febrifuge.

YARROW Essential oil, a bitter component; it is a bitter tonic, carminative, and spasmolytic.

FLAX Seeds contain mucilage, pectin, organic acids, glycoside and an enzyme; it is soothing, pain relieving and laxative.

MEADOWSWEET A glycoside, tannin, and sugar; meadowsweet is anti-rheumatic, diuretic, diaphoretic, and spasmolytic.

WHITE BRYONY A resin, a glucoside, an alkaloid; white bryony is a drastic purgative.

CARAWAY An essential oil; it is anti-spasmodic, carminative, stomachic.

SAGE An essential oil, camphor, tannin and bitter compounds; it stops perspiration, is carminative, spasmolytic, stimulating, anti-diarrheal.

ELDER An essential oil, glycosides, mucilage and tannin; it is diaphoretic, antispasmodic, and antirheumatic.

RESTHARROW An essential oil, glyco-side, and other compounds; it is diuretic.

HOP Bitter compounds; it is antibiotic, hypnotic, sedative.

VALERIAN An essential oil; it is a tranquilliser, antispasmodic and stomachic.

YELLOW GENTIAN Bitter glycosides; yellow gentian is a tonic, stomachic.

BLACKBERRY Rich in tannin; it is astringent.

WILLOW Contains glycosides and tannin; it may be taken as a tonic or a febrifuge.

WILD THYME An essential oil; it is a bitter aromatic, tonic, expectorant, antispasmodic and disinfectant.

HORSE CHESTNUT Contains saponins, tannins, a glycoside; it is anti-phlogistic, diuretic, and increases the rate of blood circulation.

MULLEIN Contains saponins; it is soothing and expectorant.

PASSION FLOWER Contains alkaloids; it is a general antispasmodic, a tranquilliser, soothing and invigorating.

BILBERRY Fruits contain tannin, organic acids, sugars and pectin; it is astringent, antidiarrhoeic, tonic and antiseptic.

BEARBERRY Contains glycosides and is disinfectant.

ARTICHOKE Contains a bitter substance, tannins and enzymes; it is choleretic and diuretic.

MALE FERN Contains acids; it is toxic and antihelminthic.

JUNIPER An essential oil, a bitter compound; it is a diuretic, a stomachic, tonic and carminative.

MISTLETOE Contains alkaloid-like substances, a saponoside; it is diuretic, cardiotonic, hypotensive; poisonous in large quantities.

14

Glossary of therapeutic and botanical terms

Allopathy conventional medicine

Analgesic a substance that relieves pain

Antidiarrheal that which combats and stops diarrhoea

Antidote that which counteracts poison

Antihelminthic vermifuge

Antiphlogistic counteracting inflammation

Antipyretic an agent counteracting fever

Antiscorbutic of use against scurvy

Antispasmodic relieving cramps

Aphrodisiac increasing sexual appetite

Asparagine a nitrogenous crystallisable compound

Astringent promotes firming and contraction of tissues

Bechic a substance that sooths a cough

Bitter compounds plant substances which taste bitter and stimulate the glands and the appetite

Carminative relieving flatulence

Choleretic stimulating bile production

Corymb inflorescence (a stem axis bearing flowers) in which the flowers rise from different points on the stem, the lower stalks being longer so that the flowers are arranged on the same plane in a flat topped or convex cluster

Demulcent soothing, mollifying, allaying irritation

Deruptive blood purifying

Diaphoretic causing perspiration

Diuretic stimulates urine production

Drastic violent purgative

Dysmenorrhoea difficult or painful menstruation

Emetic causes vomiting

Emollient reducing irritations and inflammations

Essential oils volatile oils processed from plants and containing the scent of the plant

Febrifuge counteracts fever

Glycosides sweet chemical compounds in which a simple sugar is mixed with another organic compound

Haemostatic stops the flow of blood

Hypotensive the ability to reduce blood pressure

Mucilage a gummy secretion of plants

Pharmacopoeiae publications containing lists of drugs and instructions for the production of medicines

Renal pertaining to the kidneys

Resin An aromatic vegetable product from trees and plants, exuding naturally or obtained by incision

Salicyclates bitter compounds

Saponins glycoside substances which produce a lather

Spasmolytic that which relieves and counteracts cramps

Stimulant that which temporarily stimulates nervous or muscular activity

Stomachic a gastric stimulant

Tannin astringent vegetable substance

Tonic that which stimulates or restores vigour to the body or to an individual organ

Umbel a flat-topped cluster of flowers, stalks equal in length, radiating out from a single point, like an umbrella

Vermifuge kills worms

Vulnerary promoting the healing of wounds

15

Coltsfoot

Tussilago farfara
Compositae

A common perennial weed, with creeping, underground stems, and yellow-fringed flowers appearing on scaly stems before the leaves develop. It is common throughout Europe and North Asia, especially on clay soils. It produces daisy-like flowers in March and April.

The leaves, flowers and root are used. Leaves are collected in June and July and the flower stalks in February.

All parts of the plant contain mucilage. It is demulcent (soothing), expectorant and tonic, and has been in use for centuries as one of the most popular cough mixtures. The botanical name means 'cough dispeller'. The smoking of the leaves for the relief of a cough was recommended by Dioscorides, Galen, Pliny and Boyle. The leaves are the basis of herb tobacco, other ingredients being buck bean, eyebright, betony, rosemary, thyme, lavender and camomile flowers. It is said to relieve asthma and bronchitis. In Paris coltsfoot flowers used to be painted on the doorposts of apothecaries' shops as a sign.

A decoction made of 30g (1oz) leaves in 1.25 litres (1 quart) of water, boiled down to a pint, sweetened with honey or liquorice, and taken in teacupful doses is good for colds and asthma, and an infusion of flowers and leaves has long been a country remedy for colds.

Culpepper says: 'The fresh leaves, or juice, or syrup thereof is good for a bad dry cough, or wheezing and shortness of breath,' also 'it helpeth St Anthony's Fire (erisypelis) and burnings, and is singular good to take away wheals.'

Coltsfoot 'rock' is still sold as a pleasant sweet, and it is also good for coughs.

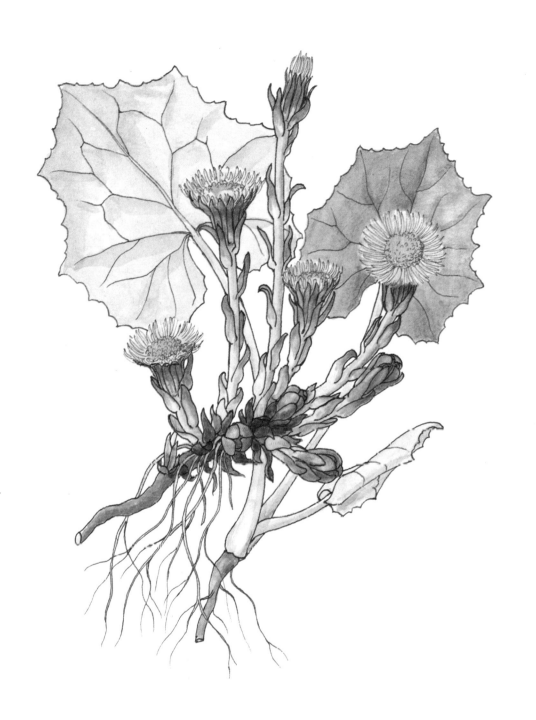

Butterbur

Petasites hybridus
Compositae

A perennial plant with a creeping underground rhizome and hollow stems, bearing groups of pinkish white flowers, butterbur grows throughout Europe on banks and in muddy alluvial soils by water. The flowers appear in February and March before the large flat, circular leaves.

The root produces an alkaloid, an essential oil, tannin and a mucilage. A tincture of this rhizome is used in homeopathy for pains in the neck and head. In herbalism the plant is recommended for its vulnerary powers and for skin conditions. The butterbur is in the same family as coltsfoot.

The name of the genus is derived from 'petasos', the Greek word for the felt hats worn by shepherds, and familiar to us from the pictures of Mercury, the messenger of the gods, who wore one decorated with wings. The leaves are large enough to make a hat. It is called butterbur possibly because the large leaves were used to wrap butter in hot weather. Historically it was said to have gained a reputation for success against the plague (Lyte 1578, 'a soveraigne medicine against the plague.') The seeds were much used for divination and charms.

The part used in medicine is the rhizome, and the medicinal action is as a heart stimulant, and as such should only be taken under advice, as a remedy in fevers, asthma, colds and urinary complaints, a decoction being taken warm. Both butterbur and coltsfoot are specific homeopathic remedies for severe neuralgia and pains in the small of the back.

Gerard: 'The roots dried and beaten to powder and drunke in wine is a soveraigne medicine against the plague and pestilent fevers . . . it killeth worms. The powder of the roots cureth all naughty filthy ulcers, if it be strewed therein.'

Culpepper: 'It is under the dominion of the Sun and therefore is a great strengthener of the heart and cheerer of the vital spirits.'

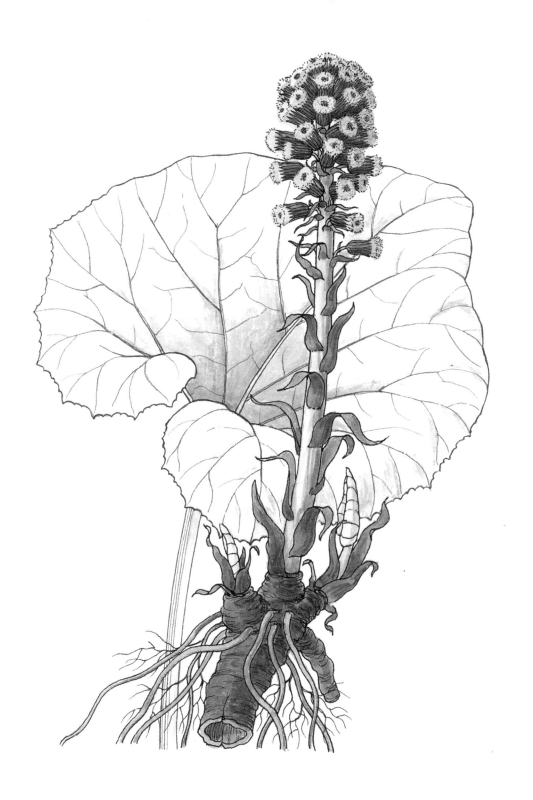

Dandelion

Taraxacum officinale
Compositae

Such a well known plant hardly needs describing, with its bright yellow flower heads and hollow stems of sticky juice growing from a rosette of indented leaves. It is a bitter tonic, diuretic, stomachic and induces the flow of bile. An infusion of the fresh root is used for gallstones, jaundice and other liver disorders. It acts as a general stimulant to the system, and is used in many medicines especially for kidney and liver disorders. The early Arabian physicians, Rhazes and Abou ben Sina (Avicenna), mention it, and the name of the genus comes from the Greek 'taraxos'—disorder and 'akos'—remedy, and the English name derives from dent de lion, from the lion's tongue leaves. Cultivated dandelion leaves, which are larger than the wild ones, are grown and sold as salad greens on the continent of Europe, and the young leaves of wild plants are eaten alone or with lettuce in the spring as a tonic, as well as a delicious food. The leaves cooked with spinach are also very beneficial. Dandelions also grow successfully in Australia.

A broth of dandelion roots, sliced, and stewed in boiling water with some leaves of sorrel and the yolk of an egg, taken daily for some months, has been known to cure chronic liver congestion. A strong decoction is useful for stones and gravel. It has a good effect in increasing the appetite, is given for dyspepsia and for promoting the digestion.

The leaves and flowers are used in summer for making dandelion tea, and the flowers for dandelion wine. Infuse 30g (1oz) dandelion in 600ml (1 pint) of boiling water for 10 minutes, sweeten with honey if desired and drink several glasses a day. For a sluggish liver take 60g (2oz) freshly sliced dandelion root, boil in 1.5 litres (2 pints) water, reduce to 600ml (1 pint) then add 30g (1oz) compound tincture of horseradish and take 60–120g (2–4oz).

As a general tonic in spring Mességué gives this recipe. Pick leaves in spring, and flowers as they come. Make a decoction or infusion by putting a good handful of roots or leaves or both into a litre (1.5 pints) of water and drink 3 cups a day.

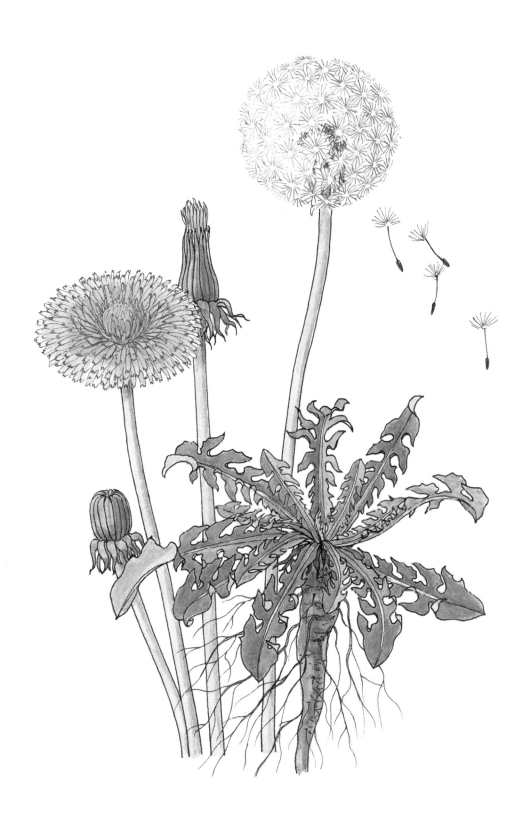

Wild Garlic

Ramson's and Bear's Garlic
Allium ursinum
Liliaceae

This is found in damp woods all over Europe, and can be planted in Australia. The leaves are like those of lily of the valley and the white flowers are in an umbel appearing from April to June. The whole plant smells of onions and has an acrid taste and cannot be substituted for cultivated garlic (*Allium sativum*). It produces an essential oil containing, among other things, vitamin C. The whole plant is used in herbalism and it has always been highly prized in folk medicine. Wild garlic has the same properties as cultivated garlic which are legion. Cultivated garlic is a plant of great antiquity. It is an antibiotic and general antiseptic, good for curing diarrhoea, for stimulating the liver, against gout, sciatica, hot flushes, hypertension and good for the circulatory system as well as being a cleanser for the whole body.

Culpeper: ' . . . a herb of Mars . . . performs almost miracles in phlegmatic habits of the body.'

A decoction consisting of a head of garlic to a litre (1.5 pints) of water or stock, to be taken 3 cupfuls a day is beneficial, and so is garlic added to the food every day in salads, curries, casseroles and soups.

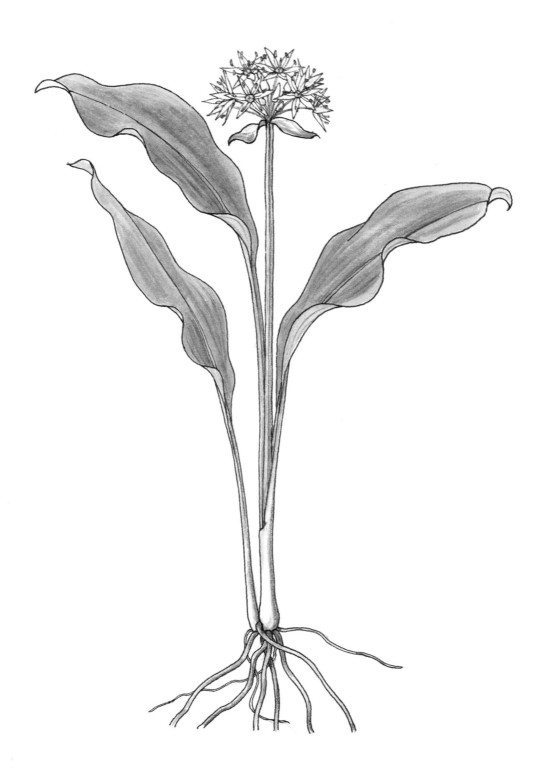

Cowslip

Primula officinalis
Primulaceae

The cowslip is found throughout Europe in dry grassland, in open woods and hedges, although, sadly, it seems to be less common in Britain than it was. The flowers are deep yellow in an umbel and smell very sweet, appearing in April and May. The plant, particularly the root, possesses, in common with other members of the primrose family, many active medical properties. It is used in homeopathy to treat neuralgias and respiratory disorders. The action is sedative and antispasmodic, and in the past was used 'to ease paines in the head,' for insomnia, to improve the memory and to remove spots and freckles from the skin.

Cowslip wine was drunk by, among others, the poet, Alexander Pope, and is a sedative and pleasantly soporific, the flowers having slightly narcotic properties. Cowslip water consisting of 0.5 kilo (1lb) freshly gathered blossom infused in 1 litre (1.5 pints) boiling water and simmered down with loaf sugar to a fine yellow syrup, taken with a little water, is beneficial for giddiness, nervous debility or excitement. In the past young cowslip leaves were often eaten in salads.

Cowslip wine: 4.5 litres (1 gallon) of yellow petals or 'peeps' with 2 kilos (4lb) loaf sugar, and the rind of 3 lemons are added to a gallon of cold water. A cup of fresh yeast is added and the mixture stirred every day for a week. It is then put into a barrel with the juice of the lemons and left to work. When fermentation stops it is corked down for 8 or 9 months and then bottled. The wine should be perfectly clear and of a pale yellow colour.

Culpeper: 'A herb of Venus, and it is under the sign Aries, and our city dames know well enough the ointment or distilled water of it adds to beauty or at least restores it when it is lost.'

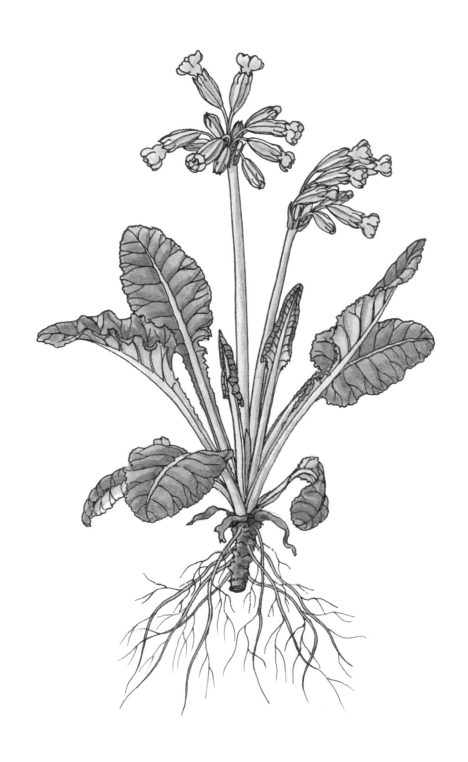

Comfrey

Symphytum officinale
Boraginaceae

A plant growing all over Europe and temperate Asia, cultivable in Australasia, comfrey is common throughout England by roads, on banks of rivers and ditches and in damp places. It is a member of the borage and forget-me-not family, a tall plant, with rough hairy leaves, and flowers in one-sided clusters. The flowers are cream, pink or purple and appear most of the summer from May onwards. Russian comfrey has rich blue flowers and was introduced into this country in the last century as a fodder plant.

Comfrey was mainly cultivated in the distant past, in gardens, as a herb for healing wounds and as a remedy for broken or dislocated bones. It was much used to treat fractures in the Middle Ages. The plant abounds in mucilage and has an emollient action, and it is used in herbal remedies against stomach upsets, lung troubles and coughs. Comfrey leaves were put round sprains, swellings and bruises either fresh or as formentations or poultices and also on severe cuts and ulcers. It has always been deemed excellent for soothing tender or inflamed places. Comfrey roots, together with roots of dandelion and chicory, make an acceptable coffee substitute.

A remedy for coughs: boil 30g (1oz) crushed root in 0.75 litre (1 pint) of water for 10 minutes, then add an equal quantity of new milk to the contents of the pan and simmer for 15 minutes. A wineglassful should be taken every 3 hours. An ordinary infusion of the hairy leaves may also be taken, flavoured with lemon juice.

Comfrey ointment works like magic on sprained backs or joints. Pills are also available in health shops.

Gerard: 'It joyeth in watery ditches, in fat and fruitful meadows.'

Culpeper: 'This is a herb of Saturn, and I suppose under the sign Capricorn: cold, dry and earthy in quality.'

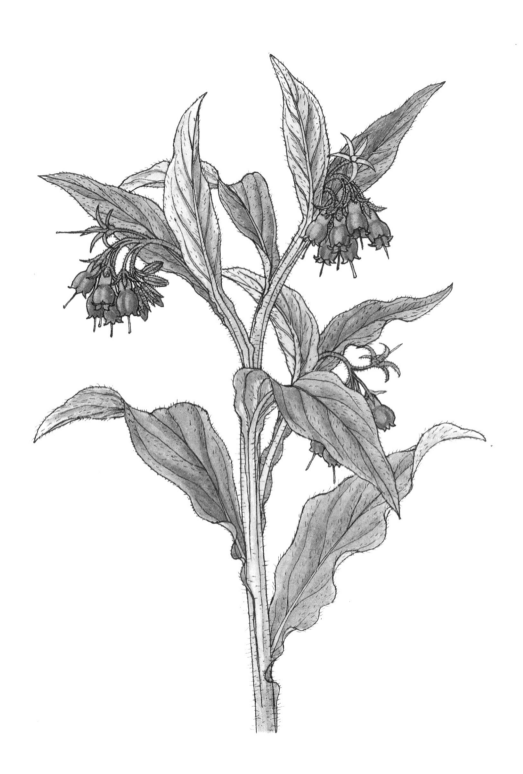

Plantain

Plantago lanceolata
Plantaginaceae

A very common plant which grows on dry soils and waste grounds all over Europe, and is found in Australasia. The flowers appear from April to October and are very small, in a dense brown or green spike. It is a weed which is a great nuisance in lawns. It is antidiarrhoeic, expectorant, emollient and vulnerary. A decoction, a syrup and an extract are made from the whole plant to treat catarrh, bronchitis and asthma. Used externally the leaves are healing for wounds. As a gargle it is good for sore throats, and as an eyewash it is prescribed for conjunctivitis and inflammation of the eyelids.

In the Highlands of Scotland the herb is called 'slanlus', a Gaelic word which means literally, 'the plant of healing', and as such it has been famed for centuries. Dioscorides advised that it should be applied as a poultice to every kind of sore, and in Sutherland, among other places, it is an accepted remedy for toothache. Culpeper said: 'the roots and pellitory beaten into powder and put into hollow teeth takes away the pains of them.' A gipsy remedy for wicklows and similar nasty places on the fingers is to soak plantain leaves in hot water and bind them round the finger. It is also as good as dock leaves for minor wounds and nettle and insect stings.

An infusion for upset stomach or piles: pour 600ml (1 pint) boiling water on 30g (1oz) of the herb, stand in a warm place for 20 minutes, strain and let cool, and take a wineglassful 3 or 4 times a day.

Shakespeare mentions plantain leaves as being excellent for broken skin in *Romeo and Juliet* and in *The Two Noble Kinsmen*, 'These poor slight sores need not a Plantain'.

Culpeper: 'This is under Venus and it cures the head by its antipathy to Mars, and the privities by its sympathy to Venus; neither is there a martial disease but it cures . . . all the Plantains are good wound herbs.'

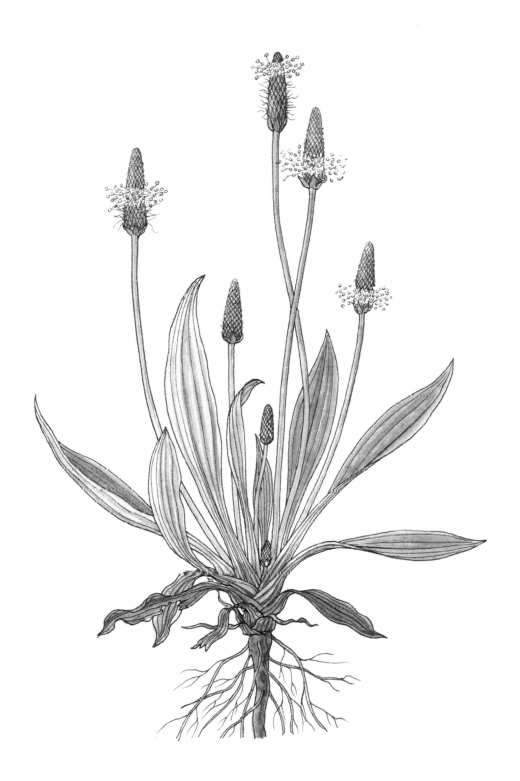

Silverweed

Potentilla anserina
Rosaceae

A perennial plant with creeping stems and silvery, silky leaves, very common on dry soils. Yellow flowers appear in July and August. It is one of the commonest Potentillas, growing from Lapland to the Azores, in Chile, Armenia and China.

Silverweed is used in homeopathy as an antispasmodic in gastritis and other similar ailments. All parts of the plant contain tannin, and in modern herbal medicine the whole herb is used, dried, for its mildly astringent and tonic action. The herb is gathered in June for drying. Historically silverweed was used to treat ulcers and sores, and was often put into shoes to keep the feet comfortable when walking long distances. Roots were eaten raw, boiled, roasted or ground into a flour. Silverweed should only be used with advice from the herbalist.

A strong infusion used as a lotion will stop the bleeding of piles; an ordinary infusion (30g/1oz to 60ml/1 pint boiling water) being taken as a medicine or, sweetened with honey, as a gargle. It is also good for stomach cramps, for the heart and the abdomen. In Europe a tablespoon of the herb, boiled in a cup of milk, was used as a remedy for tetanus. The decoction has been used for mouth ulcers, spongey gums and for fixing loose teeth. Distilled water of the herb was used as a cosmetic for removing freckles, spots and pimples, and formentations were used to prevent pitting by smallpox.

Culpeper: 'This plant is under Venus and deserves to be universally known in medicine.'

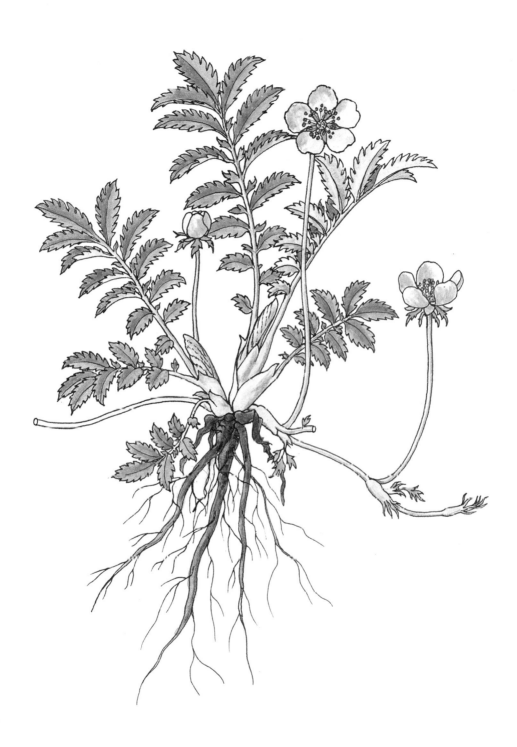

Bog Bean

Buck Bean
Meryanthes trifoliata
Gentianaceae

The bog bean is a perennial aquatic plant which is widespread throughout Europe in ponds and marshes. It has trifoliate leaves and white and pink flowers in May and June, these are above the water, the stem being submerged. Bog bean forms large patches on the surface of water. The leaves and rhizome contain bitter compounds, and the plant is stomachic, tonic and sedative. The leaves are the parts of the plant which are most used, being collected from April to June.

The bog bean is used as a bitter tonic in the same way as yellow gentian. An infusion of the leaves acts against liver deficiencies and soothes digestive troubles. In ancient times the plant was held to be of great value against scurvy. An extract is made from the leaves as a tonic which is given in cases of rheumatism and in skin diseases. An infusion of 30g (1oz) of the dried herb in 600ml (1 pint) water is taken by the cupful. Buck bean tea, the infusion, is said to cure dyspepsia and a torpid liver due to its tonic qualities. It can be taken alone or mixed with wormwood, centaury or sage. It is also used as a sedative, often with water mint and valerian.

The bitterness of the buck bean has led to its use as a substitute for hops in brewing beer. In modern herbal practice it is considered a most valuable tonic, aiding digestion and restoring strength.

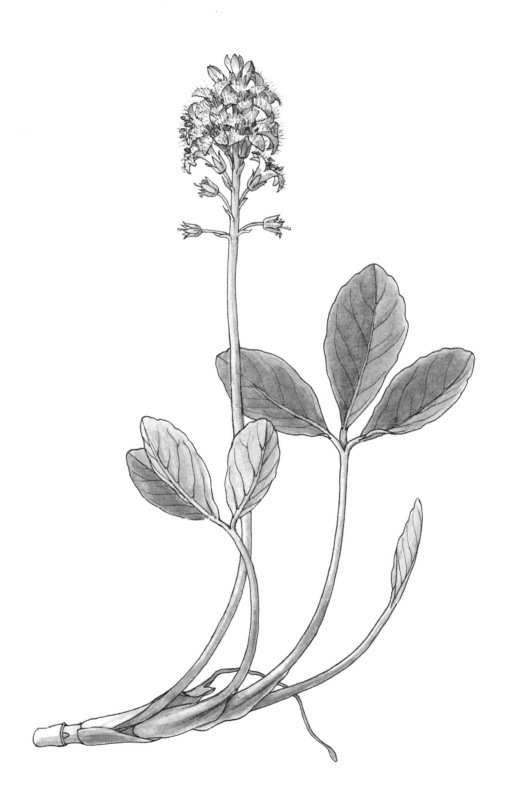

Silver birch

Betula pendula
Betulaceae

A small, delicate tree with papery white bark common in Europe and North Asia in cool woods and on damp soils. The young leaves are rich in saponins, they are diuretic and help the heart.

The birch is used in various ways, as an infusion, oil or extract, to treat urinary disorders, in herbalism to treat some skin complaints, and in the cosmetic industry in lotions and creams. The scent known as russian leather is produced by treating skins with a birch pitch or tar, and books bound in russian leather are not liable to become mouldy.

The young shoots and leaves secrete a resinous, acid substance which, combined with alkaloids, is said to be a tonic laxative. The leaves which have an aromatic scent and a bitter taste are used in the form of an infusion (birch tea) for gout, rheumatism, dropsy and kidney stones. Mességué gives several recipes for silver birch remedies.

(1) Infusion of leaves: a small handful of fresh leaves in a litre of water to be taken in 3 cupfuls a day, as a diuretic.

(2) Half a handful of fresh leaves to each litre of water in a bath for slimming.

(3) For a foot or hand bath for rheumatism or gout: 4–6 handfuls of chopped bark in a bowl of water, let it stand for half an hour, heat and use twice a day.

(4) Tea for colds: 15 pinches of the dried leaves, 10 pinches of wild pansy flowers and lime flowers in a litre of water. Take 3 or 4 cupfuls a day.

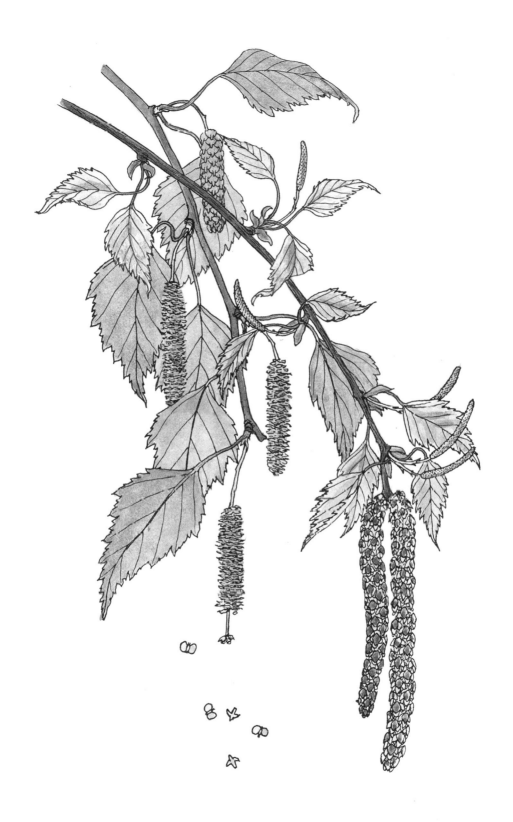

Soapwort

Bouncing Bet, Latherwort, Fuller's herb, Bruisewort
Saponaria officinalis
Caryophylaceae

A perennial plant with large clusters of pink flowers and an underground rhizome, common on banks and roadsides all over Europe, growing 60cm (24in) high. This plant contains a saponin and the leaves contain vitamin C. It is expectorant, diuretic and purgative and the leaves and roots can be used as detergents. The rhizome is used as a decoction to treat respiratory infections and is also effective for boils and dermatitis.

Soapwort was used extensively in ancient Greece. It grows well in English gardens. Due to its saponin content it must be **very cautiously used** but as a purifier of the blood it has great value, and has proved useful in jaundice and venereal complaints. Skin diseases, boils and abcesses have been cured by an infusion of soapwort taken over a long period. (Infusion: 60g (2oz) leaves to 600ml (1 pint) water, a glassful taken 4 times a day.) In France and Germany a decoction of the root is given internally in cases of gout, rheumatism and similar disorders.

The plant is known as soapwort because when the leaves are boiled in water a strong lather is produced, and in ancient times this herb was a substitute for soap, used by the mendicant friars. This lather removes grease and stains. In the Middle Ages it was also used in brewing, because adding the root to the beer produced a good 'head'. The dried herb can be obtained from any good herbalist, but when taking the fluid great care must be taken to keep to the exact dose.

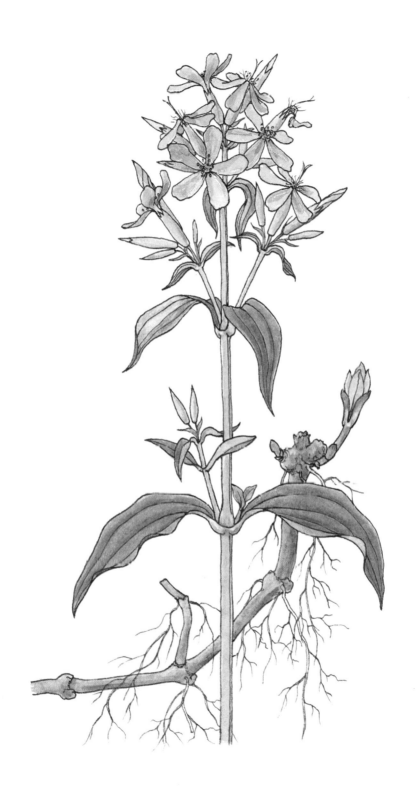

Sanicle

Sanicula europea
Umbellifereae

An umbelliferous perennial, sanicle is common in deciduous woods and thickets, and damp, moist places particularly on chalky soil, growing in the British Isles, central and northern Europe and the mountains of tropical Africa. It is 40cm (16in) high and flowers from May to July.

The leaves and rhizome contain saponins, tannin, a bitter compound and an essence. It is mainly used as a vulnerary for septic wounds and as a gargle. Formerly official, sanicle is still used in remote parts of Europe to treat internal haemorrhages. It was very popular in the Middle Ages and the origin of the name explains why, it is from the Latin word 'sano', meaning I heal, or I cure. The whole herb is collected in June and dried, gathered like all herbs on a fine day in the morning when the dew has dried.

Sanicle is usually given in a combination with other herbs in the treatment of blood disorders. It is said to clear the blood of morbid secretions and to leave it healthier and in better condition. The infusion of 30g (1oz) to 600ml (1 pint) boiling water is taken in wineglassful doses. It is used as a gargle for sore throats and quinsy (tonsilitis), and whenever an astringent gargle is needed, and it is particularly popular in France and Germany.

Culpeper: 'Mars owns this herb . . . there is not found any herb that can give such present help to man or beast, when the disease falls on the lungs and throat . . . gargling with a decoction of the leaves and roots made in water, and a little honey put thereto.'

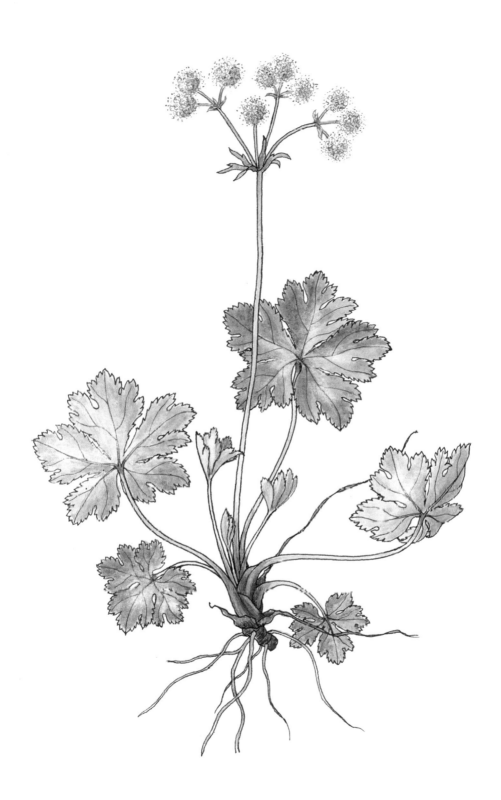

Alder Buckthorn

Black Dogwood
Frangula alnus
Ranunculaceae

This is a thornless shrub or small tree, with small flowers that turn into red or dark purple fruits. It is widespread throughout Europe and western Asia, growing in scrub and at the edge of bogs in sandy soils. It flowers in May and June. The bark and young branches contain glyocides and a laxative. A fluid extract from the bark is a recognised remedy in both the British and United States pharmacopoeia as an aperient, like cascara.

The bark and leaves yield a yellow die, the unripe berries give a good green and the ripe ones a blue/grey die, so alder buckthorn is of interest to home weavers. The wood of the shrub is used to give charcoal which is much preferred to that from other trees by gunpowder makers, and, indeed the German name for this plant is pulverholz or powder wood.

The medical action of alder buckthorn is tonic, laxative and cathartic, and it is used as a gentle purgative in cases of chronic constipation, administered as a fluid extract. A decoction of the young bark is given 3 or 4 times a day made with 30g (1oz) of bark in 3.25 litres (1 quart) of water boiled down to 600ml (1 pint), but only under a doctor's advice.

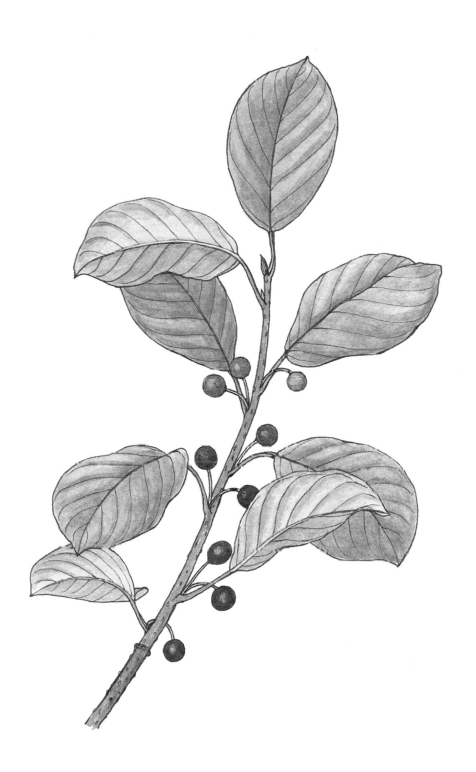

Herb Robert

Geranium robertium
Geraniaceae

A very common weed throughout Europe, Asia and north Africa, in rocky soils, woods, hedges, garden walls and stony places, often appearing in gardens. It is an annual plant 14–40cm (5.5–15.5in) high with red hairy stems and leaves and small pink flowers. The whole plant has a strong, rather unpleasant smell. Herb Robert contains a bitter compound, tannin and an essential oil, and it is astringent and sedative.

It used to be a recognised remedy but is now only used in herbalism to treat eye conditions, skin eruptions, herpes and oral inflammations. It is administered as an infusion or as compresses made from the crushed fresh plant.

Culpeper: 'Under the dominion of Venus, commended against the stone and to stay blood.'

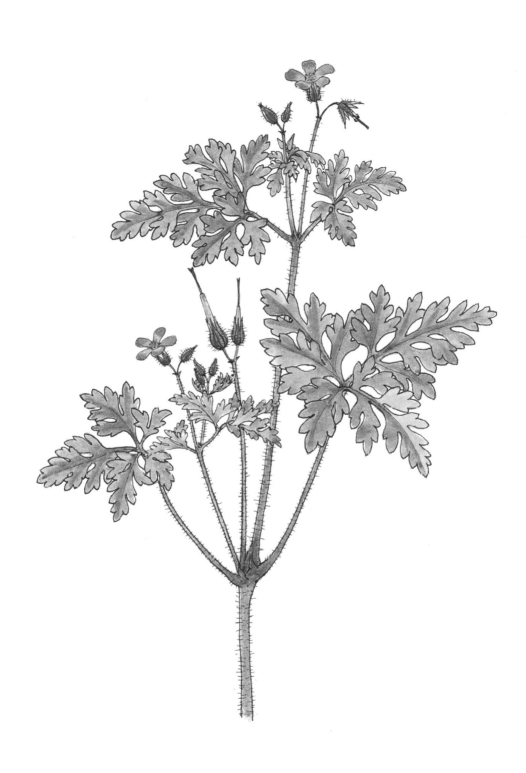

Tormentil

Potentilla erecta
Roseaceae

Tormentil is a low spreading perennial, very common, particularly on acid soils where it is damp, throughout Europe. The flowers are yellow and four petaled and appear from May to August. The rhizome contains up to 20% tannin, and it is a powerful astringent and antidiarrhoeic. It can be used as a decoction or as a tincture, and as a gargle. The decoction is used to treat haemorrhage and diarrhoea, but only under advice.

The roots used to be boiled in milk to treat stomach upsets in children and calves. They were also used, especially in the north, as a substitute for oak bark in tanning and to make a red dye. The whole plant is very astringent, considered one of the safest and most powerful of our native aromatic astringents, and for its tonic properties has been called the English sarsaparilla. There is a big demand for the rhizome which is still used in modern herbal medicine for diarrhoea and as a gargle for sore throats. The fluid extract is also applied to cuts and wounds. A decoction is recommended for piles and inflamed eyes, which is made by boiling 60g (2oz) of the bruised root in 1.5 litres (2.5 pints) of water until reduced by a third. This is also said to make warts disappear. A simple infusion is made by scalding 30g (1oz) powdered tormentil with 600ml (1 pint) water and taking as required in wineglassful doses, and this is good for stomach upsets.

Tormentil was historically used to cure ague, smallpox and whooping cough, and was also given for cholera and as a lotion for ulcers, in short a cure-all.

Culpeper: 'This is a herb of the sun . . . it resisteth putrefaction.'

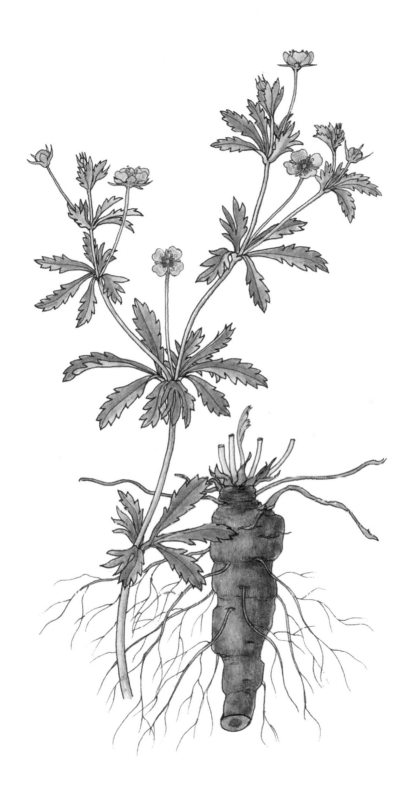

Stinging Nettle

Uticaria dioica
Uticaceae

A very well known and common perennial weed, growing to 1 metre (3ft) or more; stinging nettles show the presence of good soil rich in nitrogen. They grow in Europe and Asia, Japan, South Africa, Australia and the Andes. The leaves have stinging hairs which contain a venom causing irritation and inflammation. They also attract a number of butterflies which lay their eggs on nettles.

The fibre of the stems is similar to that of hemp or flax and it was used for making cloth, varying from that of the finest texture to the coarsest such as sailcloth, sacking and cordage. In Hans Andersen's story of *The Princess and the Swan Princes*, the princess weaves the swans' clothes of nettle, all except the youngest whose coat she could not finish in time and who therefore always had one wing and one arm. In Scotland nettle fibres were used as recently as the 16th century for weaving household linen. You would eat nettles, sleep in nettle sheets and dine off nettle tablecloths. Nettle cloth was held by many to last longer than linen cloth woven from flax. The twine was stronger than flax and therefore particularly useful for making fishing nets. It was used for clothing in Germany during the First World War.

The nettle has long been used as a pot herb because it is a healthy vegetable easily digested. Young shoots are cooked and eaten like spinach. (Gloves should be worn when picking them however.) They are washed in running water and cooked with the lid on for 20 minutes, then they are chopped, sieved, and warmed up in the pan with butter. In Scotland early nettles were forced under glass cloches.

The leaves are used medicinally as a decoction or infusion and in many diuretic tisanes. In homeopathy an extract of the fresh leaves is used for eczema, dysmenorrhoea and nosebleeds. Nettle is also used in lotions to make the hair grow. The whole plant may be used as a rub to treat rheumatism; this is said to be effective though doubtless painful. Nettle is antiscorbutic and nettle tea is still a common spring medicine in many rural districts, and is a good blood purifier. Water in which nettles have been boiled is said to clear the complexion of blemishes and to brighten the eyes.

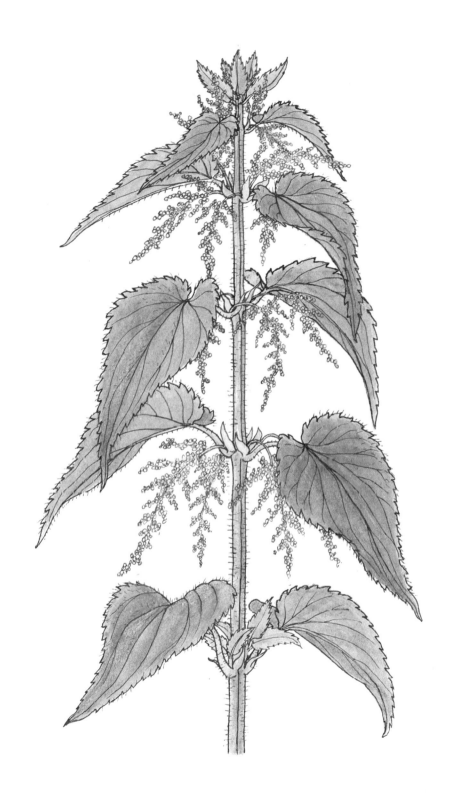

Hawthorn

May
Crataegus oxyacantha
Rosaceae

Hawthorn grows as spiny trees or bushes common in woods and hedgerows, with sweet-smelling flowers in clusters which turn into red berry-like fruit—the 'haws'. It flowers in May and June.

Hawthorn is a strong cardiac tonic which helps in the treatment of both high and low blood pressure. It is antispasmodic and sedative and is also used in the treatment of insomnia. The parts used are the dried haws and the flowers. The German name which means 'hedgethorn' shows that from early times this tree has been used as a hedge to divide fields and plots, and the word haw is an old word for 'hedge'. The therapeutic value of the hawthorn was not fully appreciated until recently although Dioscorides had mentioned it.

The medical action is cardiac, diuretic, astringent and tonic, it is said to prevent arteriosclerosis and to have a beneficial effect on the blood vessels generally. An infusion is made by using 2 tablespoons of the flowers in a cup of boiling water. The leaves have been used as an adulterant for tea, and a liqueur is made from the haws with brandy.

Mességué says that hawthorn was recommended by medical authorities in the Middle Ages and earlier as a remedy for gout, haemorrhage and pleurisy. He uses it as a tranquilliser, for those who are exhausted, lack energy, sleep badly and suffer from anxiety, and for people with high blood pressure. As hypertension has increased in recent years as a result of unhealthy food, stress and pollution, Mességué recommends it to people who suffer from heart attacks and wish to protect themselves against cholesterol and hardening of the arteries.

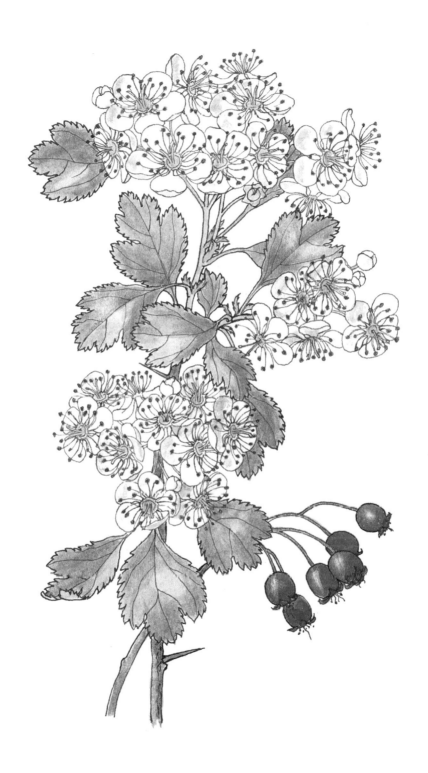

Heartsease

Wild Pansy
Viola tricolor
Violaceae

A very common annual plant on waste ground and in cultivated fields, heartsease flowers all the summer, producing yellow and purple blooms. It grows all over Europe, in northern Asia and North America.

The whole plant is used medicinally, collected from the wild and dried. It is diuretic, expectorant, depurative and laxative. It is a recognised treatment for skin erruptions and diarrhoea. It is administered as an infusion and has been used since the 16th century.

Another name for this pretty plant is 'love in idleness', and in ancient times it was much used for its potency in love charms, and as such it plays an important part in *A Midsummer Night's Dream* as a love potion. The French name is 'pensécs' meaning 'thoughts', hence our name pansy, and the saying, 'Here's Pansies, that's for thoughts' in *Hamlet*.

In the past this plant has been used for epilepsy, asthma and for diseases of the heart, which gave it its other name—'heartsease'. On the Continent the herbaceous parts of the plant have been used for their mucilaginous, demulcent and expectorant qualities.

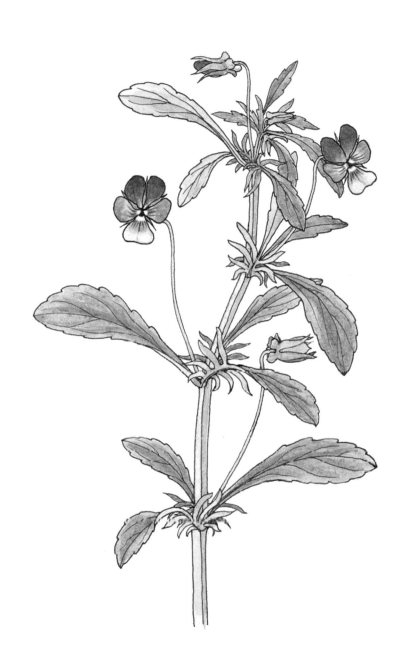

Horsetail

Equisetum arvense
Equisetaceae

Horsetails are ancient plants, allied to the ferns, large versions of which probably formed a part of the vegetation during the Carboniferous period. They look like small versions of prehistoric trees. They are chiefly distributed in temperate northern regions, growing in cultivated ground, stony and dry places and by roads particularly by water or ditches. The stems are erect with thin branches, and are decorative, but horsetail is a most invasive weed.

There is silica in the stems and bunches of them used to be sold for scouring metal, even being imported from Holland for this purpose, and the plant was also used by fletchers for finishing off their arrow shafts, by dairy maids for scouring pails and churns, and by furniture makers for rubbing down pieces of furniture. Gerard tells us that it was used for cleaning pewter and wooden utensils, and thus another name is pewterwort.

The stems are used medicinally either fresh or dried, and a fluid extract is made from them. Horsetail is diuretic and astringent; and in homeopathy a tincture of the fresh plant is administered for cystitis, anurensis and pulmonary tuberculosis. In folk medicine it is used as a gargle and mouthwash, and has been found beneficial in dropsy and kidney troubles.

Culpeper: 'There are many kinds of this herb which are but knotted rushes . . . it belongs to Saturn.' Culpeper also quotes Galen, saying it will heal sinews, and recommends it against nose bleeds, a use to which it is still put by country people.

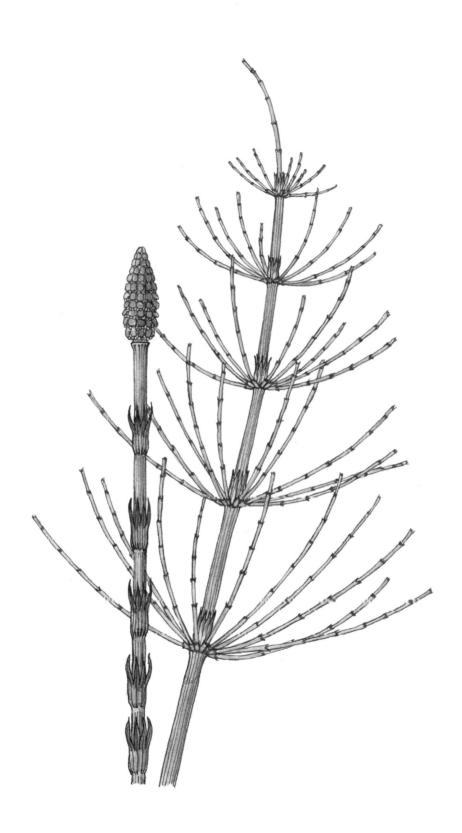

Greater Celandine

Chelidonium majus
Papaveraceae

A pretty herbaceous perennial, common throughout Europe in hedgerows and walls, and widespread near gardens, celandine is **extremely poisonous.** The flowers appear from May to July and are bright yellow.

Celandine is a strong poison and is used in homeopathy in weak doses, but is prescribed by Mességué, who is a herbalist, for external use only. It is toxic and narcotic, purgative and choleretic. A tincture of the fresh root is used for liver disorders, gastro-enteritis, pleurisy and rheumatism.

Celandine was grown as a drug in the Middle Ages and it is mentioned by Pliny. The name comes from chelidon, a swallow, as these birds were believed to take some of the yellow sap to their nestlings to protect them from blindness, or perhaps because the flowers open when the swallows first arrive and die when they go. The acrid juice was used to remove films from the cornea, as Gerard says: 'The juice of the herb is good to sharpen the sight, for it clenseth and consumeth away slimie things that cleave about the ball of the eye.' The bitter juice is used to cure warts and corns but must not come into contact with healthy skin.

Alchemists used celandine in their search for the philosopher's stone, and called it 'coeli donum', gift of heaven. This is one of the herbs which it is absolutely essential to treat with care. Mességué uses it for rheumatism, gout, kidney trouble, insomnia, asthma, bronchitis, but only *externally*.

Culpeper: 'This is a herb of the Sun, and under the celestial lion, and is one of the best cures for the eyes.'

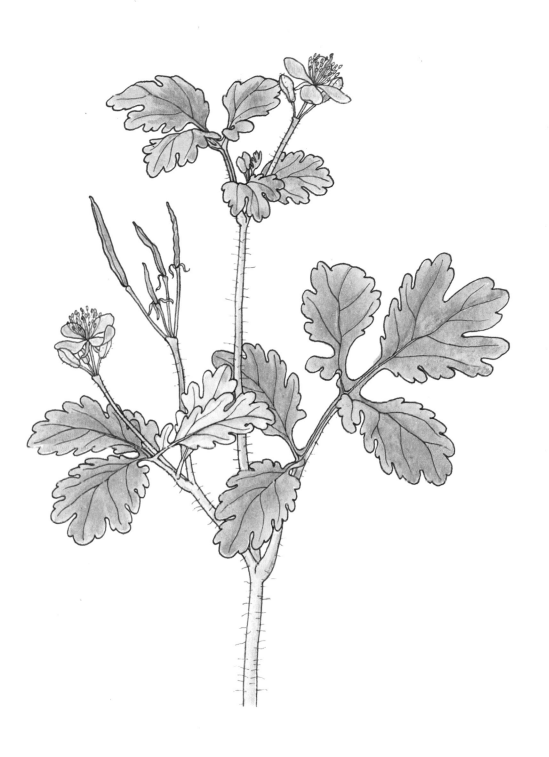

Lime

Tilia cordata
Tiliaceae

Lime is a common straight-trunked tree growing to 50 metres (130ft), flowering in June and July and scenting the whole neighbourhood. It is common in Europe and will also grow in Australia. The flowers contain an essential oil, and they are used in infusions to treat respiratory catarrh and as antispasmodics, or simply as a delicious and refreshing tea or tisane. It is particularly popular in France where the tisane is called 'tilleul'.

Lime flowers are used as an infusion and there is no better guarantee for a good night's sleep than a cup of lime tea, particularly in cases of insomnia, nerves, for the very old and the very young. It is mildly diuretic and therefore good for gout and rheumatism.

The tea: Take a good handful of flowers to a litre of water, 3 cups during the day and a cup at bedtime.

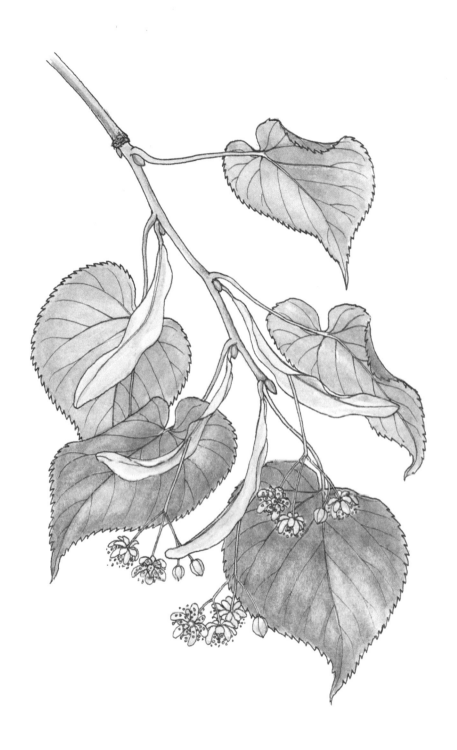

Lady's Mantle

Alchemilla vulgaris
Roseceae

A graceful perennial, lady's mantle is common all over Europe and is cultivable in Australia. In Great Britain it is mainly found in the colder districts growing on high ground such as the Scottish Highlands and the Yorkshire Dales. The leaves are scalloped and toothed, and the flowers, in bloom from June to August, are numerous and tiny, forming in clouds, yellow-green in colour.

The plant contains tannin, and is tonic, astringent and deruptive. It is used in cases of loss of appetite, intestinal complaints, and to help the menstrual cycle. The whole herb is gathered in June and July and dried. For internal use an infusion of 20g (0.75oz) of the dried plant to 1 litre (1.75 pint) water, is given.

The name comes from the fact that in the Middle Ages the plant was identified with the Virgin Mary. The generic name, *Alchemilla* is derived from the Arabic word, alkemelych meaning alchemy, because of the amazing powers of the plant. It was thought that the virtues lay in the influence the plant had on the dew drops lying on its leaves, these dew drops being part of many magic potions. In fact it is still believed by many that the drops are exuded by the leaves themselves. They were one of the substances used by the alchemists in their mixtures for attempting to make base metals into gold.

In modern herbal treatment lady's mantle is used in cases of excessive menstruation and in all 'ladies' troubles'.

Culpeper: 'Helps women who have over flagging breasts, causing them to grow less hard, both when drunk and outwardly applied.'

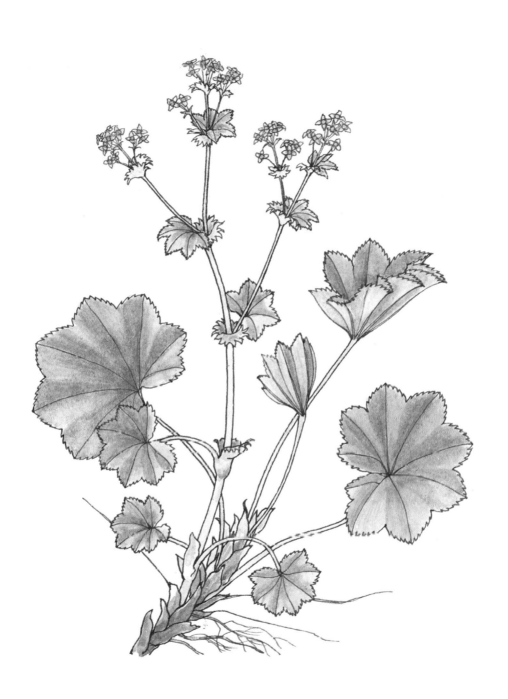

Mallow

Malva sylvestris
Malvaceae

A common perennial, growing all over Europe, on the edges of fields, on banks and in hedges. The flowers are pink-purple with five petals and bloom from June to August.

The plant contains mucilage, particularly in the leaves and flowers. The leaves contain traces of vitamin A, B, B2 and C. It is soothing, pectoral, mildly astringent and an intestinal stimulant. It is used internally as an infusion for digestive and urinary disorders, and externally as a decoction for bathing and as a gargle. The mallow has been used medicinally since 700 BC.

The boiled leaves make a wholesome vegetable. It was once commonly used as a soup, and the ancient Greeks and Romans made great use of mallows as medicinal plants. The poet Horace informed everybody that he lived on olives, chicory and mallow. St Hildegarde in the 12th century recommended it for many maladies including drowsiness, headaches, diseases of the kidneys and poisoning. 16th century doctors said that, 'Whoever drank a potion of mallow every morning was guaranteed protection against any disease for that whole day.' Mallow has more soothing properties than any other plant, and in infusions, decoctions, lotions and compresses and eye baths it has a soothing effect. It is also a good remedy for constipation.

Pick the leaves and the flowers just before they are in full bloom, and dry them quickly in shade in a well aired place. The flower centres, sometimes called 'fairy cheeses' can be eaten, or you can collect them as they are the seed cases and sow the seeds.

An infusion: 15 pinches of flowers or 20 pinches of leaves to a litre (1.5 pints) of water, take 3 or 4 cups a day. This is a good digestive.

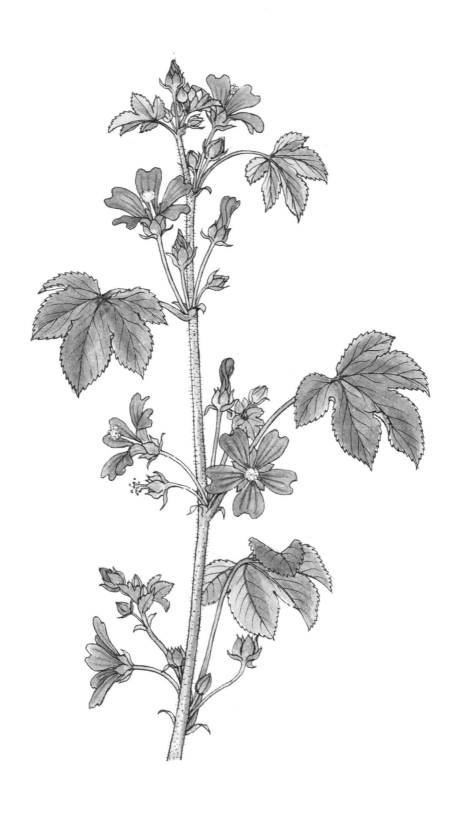

Arnica

Arnica montana
Compositae

A perennial herb growing in central and southern Europe, arnica grows in woods and mountain pastures in acid soil. The leaves form a flat rosette from which rises the flower stalk 20–60cm (8–24in) high with bright orange-yellow 'daisy' flowers. It has been found wild in England and Scotland but this is really a cultivated plant. It can be sown in gardens (sow in spring and plant out in May), or propogated by root division.

The flowers heads (*Flor. Arnicae*) and tinctures of the flowers and the roots (*Tinct. Arnicae*) are used medicinally. Arnica stimulates the circulation, and is hypertensive; it must be heavily diluted before use. In folk medicine the plant has been used to treat a wide variety of illnesses and as an abortive.

It has an irritant action on the stomach with its stimulant and diuretic effect, and **great care must be taken** as some people are sensitive to arnica. Many severe cases of poisoning have resulted from taking it internally.

The tincture is chiefly used as an application to bruises and wounds, hence its name 'the tumbler's cure all'.

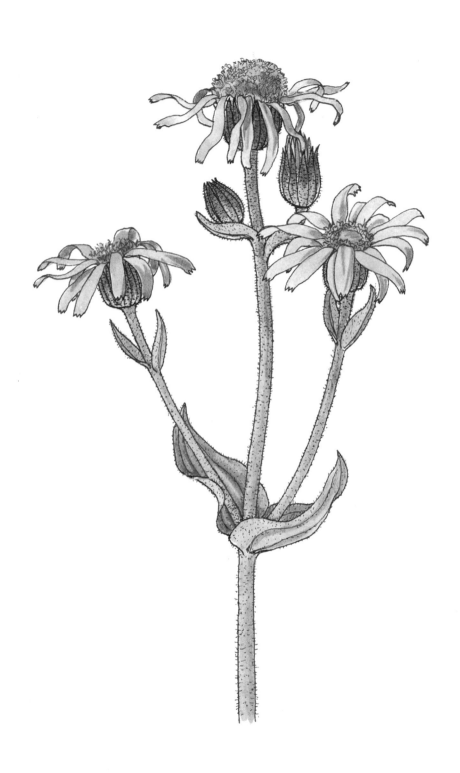

Camomile

Wild Camomile
Mactricaria chamomilla
Compositae

This is an aromatic annual weed with small flowers like daisies widespread throughout Europe. The blue essence produced from the flowers (*Ol. Chamomillae*) is used for treating inflammations and allergies, it is carminative, stomachic, vulnary, sedative and tonic. An infusion of the flowers (*Flores Chamomillae*) is used to treat a large variety of ills, particularly as a nerve sedative and a tonic (15g/0.5oz dried flowers to 600ml/1 pint water). Wild camomile is the version illustrated here, but common camomile (see below) is also interesting.

Common Camomile or Roman Camomile
Anthemis nobilis
Compositae
A common creeping plant growing all over western and southern Europe and wild in Great Britain, it has finely divided leaves and perfumed, conical white flowers from July to September. Common camomile looks like a small marguerite. The plant produces an essential oil (*Ol. Chamomill. Roman.*) and is antispasmodic, tonic and stomachic.

An infusion of the fresh plant is used for migraines, neuralgia and nervous sickness. Used externally as a decoction it is effective in treating ulcers, wounds and conjunctivitis. It is one of the oldest herbs; the Egyptians held it in great esteem and dedicated it to the gods, and no plant was better known to country people. All herbals included it, agreeing that camomile needed no description, having been grown for centuries in English gardens for use as a common domestic medicine. It will also grow in other parts of the world.

It is aromatic, with a scent of apples, and this scent is given out when it is walked on, so it was a strewing herb for floors and cultivated as a lawn plant. Camomile is known as 'the plants' physician' as it is said to improve all the other plants growing in the same garden. The double or cultivated varieties are those in the British pharmacopoeia and these are easily grown from seed. An infusion of 30g (1oz) flowers to 600ml (1 pint) boiling water (camomile tea) is soothing and sedative and absolutely harmless. It is also delicious.

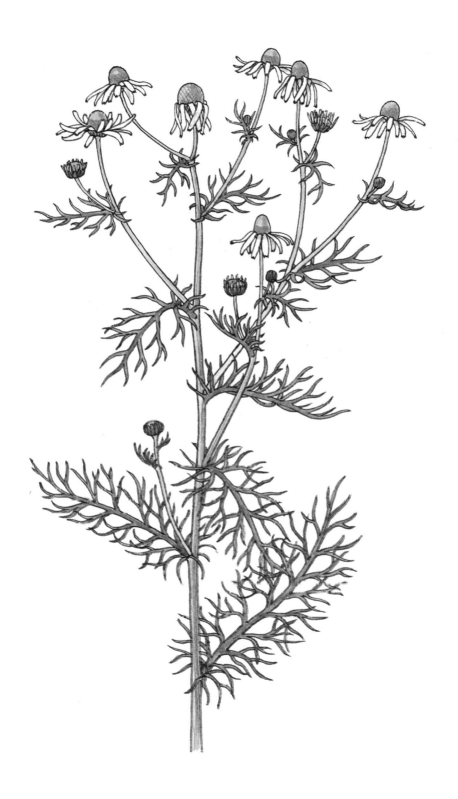

Rosemary

Rosmarinus officinalis
Labiatae

A highly aromatic shrub which grows wild round the Mediterranean, but rosemary can be grown successfully in gardens anywhere in a sunny, sheltered place. It may be grown from seed but roots quickly from cuttings taken in August; it likes a light soil and a south aspect. The small pale blue flowers appear from May to July and it is then that small sprigs should be removed for drying as the scent is strongest at that time.

The leaves and flowers produce an essential oil which is an excellent stimulant and antispasmodic. Herbal remedies recommend an infusion of the leaves; it is also used for rheumatism in baths, as a gargle and in shampoos and hair tonics. It is a soporific drink at bedtime, and of course as everyone knows it is an essential herb in cooking, especially for lamb and fish.

In ancient Greece and Rome the plant was revered. It had the reputation of strengthening the memory, hence 'rosemary for remembrance', and became a symbol of fidelity, being worn in bridal wreaths and bouquets. No medieval garden was without it; rosemary was a strewing herb for floors, and used as incense. Greek students wore it to help the brain ('It helpeth the brain, strengthening the memory, and is very medicinable for the head', Hacket 1607). Although a hot-country herb, like lavender, rosemary grows particularly well in this country. Sir Thomas More let it 'runn all over my garden walls, not only because my bees love it, but because it is a herb sacred to remembrance, and therefore, to friendship.'

It is tonic and astringent; oil of rosemary has carminative properties, and is good for stomach and nerves, curing many cases of headache. It is used externally for the hair and scalp, and as a bath additive, it improves the skin. It is said to help gout and rheumatism and to keep you looking young. As well as all this rosemary has long been considered a safeguard from witches and all evil influences, and sprigs under the pillow protect the sleeper from bad dreams. When used in cooking it not only imparts the delicious flavour but helps the digestion, neuralgic pains and stimulates the circulation.

66

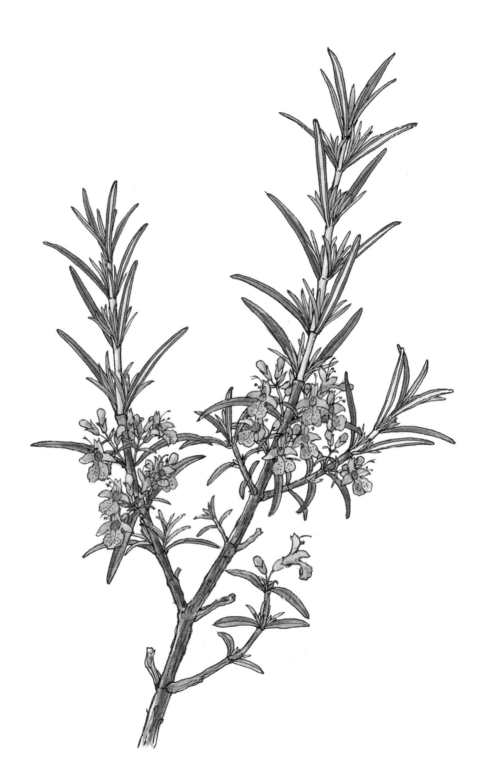

Shepherd's Purse

Capsella bursa pastoris
Crucifereae

This familiar weed with heart or purse-shaped seed pods is common throughout the world. It flowers all the year.

In modern herbal medicine the whole plant is used, dried, and given as an infusion or fluid extract, and a homeopathic tincture is made from the fresh plant. In the Middle Ages it was chiefly used as a 'blood herb' as it could stop bleeding better than any other plant. It is still used for open wounds and haemorrhages by herbalists, particularly for heavy menstrual bleeding, and is considered beneficial in some cases during the menopause. It was given to sufferers from dropsy and kidney complaints. It was also said, particularly in the New World, that a few leaves added to cabbage dishes greatly improved the flavour. It is now only used and dispensed by herbalists.

Culpeper: 'It is under the dominion of Saturn, and of a cold, dry, binding nature.'

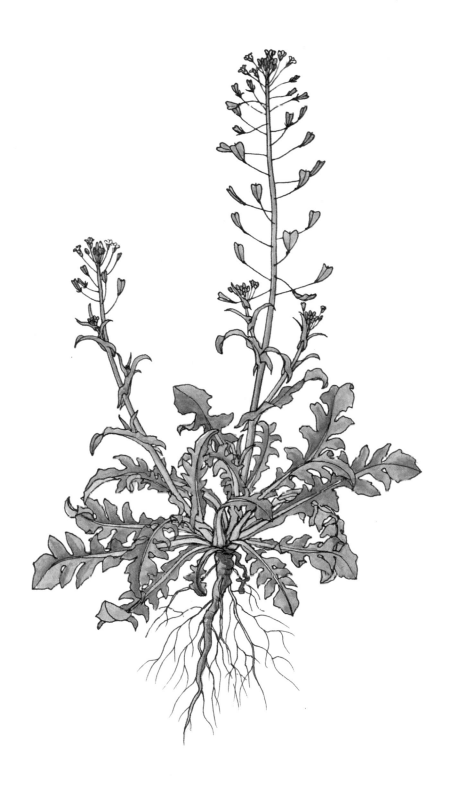

Marigold

Calendula officinalis
Compositeae

Marigold is a well-known and loved annual garden flower, originally from Egypt and cultivated in European gardens since the 12th century. It can also be grown in Australasia. The flowers are bright orange or yellow, single or double, and the garden varieties have more petals. As well as being grown for their decorative value marigolds were grown in the vegetable garden for use in broths and cakes.

A book of 1699 says the dried flowers were used to strengthen the heart, and they were much used in times of plague — particularly in broths and soups: 'In some grocers or spice-sellers houses are to be found barrels filled with them (petals) and retailed by the penny more or lesse, insomuch that no broths are well made without dried marigolds.' They were Shakespeare's 'Mary Buds' which oped their golden eyes when 'Phoebus gins arise'.

Both the leaves and the flowers are used, gathered in fine weather in the morning when the dew has dried. In the past marigold was much used as a wound ointment since it has a similar effect to that of witch hazel. The flower heads produce an essential oil which is antiphlogistic, and a vulnerary which encourages wound healing. The flowers were much used in salads and as a substitute for saffron, particularly with rice. A tea made from marigold petals is soothing for intestinal conditions, and the petals are used in buns, cakes, omelettes and puddings as they both colour and flavour the food.

Gerard: 'The floures and leaves of Marigolds being distilled, and the water dropt into red and watery eies, ceaseth the inflammation and taketh away the pain.'

Culpeper: 'A herb of the Sun and under Leo. They strengthen the heart exceedingly.'

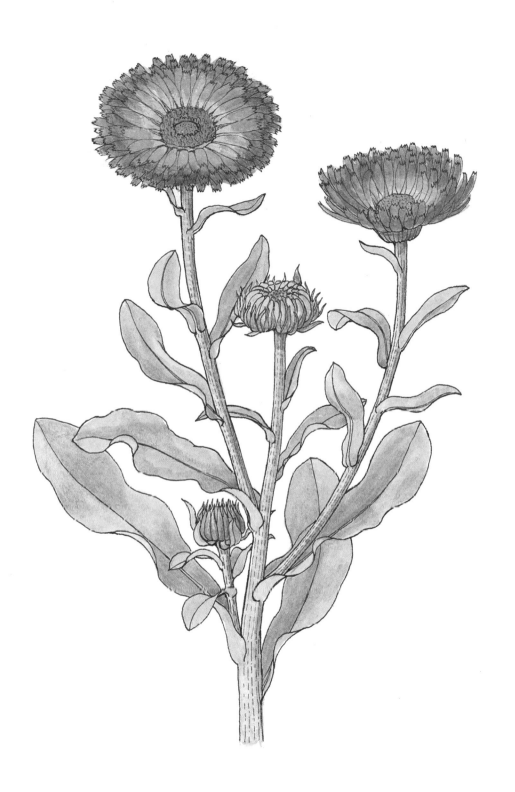

Masterwort

Peucedanum ostruthium
Umbellifereae

A plant related to dill and fennel, growing in moist meadows, masterwort is rather rare in Great Britain. It was formerly cultivated for use as a pot herb and as a medicine. It is found in mountainous regions, in cool ravines and humid gorges. Masterwort is a perennial with a stout grooved stem and dark green leaves somewhat like angelica, sometimes found in north England and Scotland, most likely as garden escapes, as this plant is a native of central Europe.

The root is the part used as it contains an essential oil which is diuretic, diaphoretic and stomachic. It was formally official but is now only used in homeopathy, as a tincture, for stomach ailments and for dermatitis. It is a stimulant, carminative, antispasmodic, and of use in treating asthma, dyspepsia and menstrual complaints.

Culpeper mentions it: 'It grows in gardens with us in England —It is a herb of Mars—The root is of a cordial sudorific nature and stands high as a remedy of great efficace in malignant and persistant fevers.' He also states that masterwort was used to treat dropsy, cramp, falling sickness, kidney and uterine troubles and gout. 'Very available in cold griefs and diseases both of the stomach and body.'

This herb is a member of the Umbellifer family, many of which are **poisonous**. It is advisable not to go looking for it and using the root, but to take it only from a homeopath or herbalist.

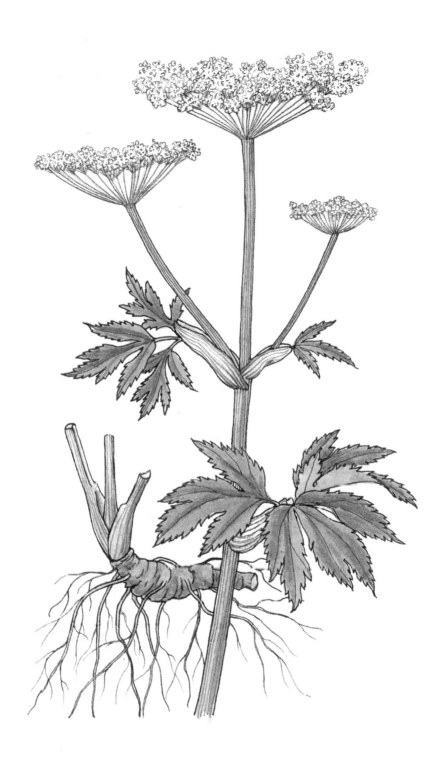

Peppermint

Mentha piperita
Labiatae

This must be about the best known herb of all as far as taste goes. It is a widely cultivated hybrid between water mint (*Mentha aquatica*) and spear mint (*Mentha spicta*), and is found locally by streams and in damp waste places. The reddish-green stems carry long, only slightly hairy leaves with short stalks, and long spikes of lilac flowers. It is found throughout Europe but is not a common native plant in Britain. It is cultivable in Australasia. Of all the members of the large mint family the varieties of peppermint are probably the most important, cultivated for years as the source of the volatile oil of peppermint which is used as a flavouring in medicines and sweets. This oil contains a large percentage of menthol which is a refreshing aromatic. Mint is antispasmodic, carminative, tonic, stimulant, excitant, and, in large quantities, aphrodisiac. An infusion produced from the leaves, and the oil in solution, has a variety of uses, for nervousness, insommnia, cramps, dizzyness, nervous sickness, spasmodic coughs and migraines. It is also used in the making of liqueurs and syrups.

Pliny tells us that the Greeks and Romans crowned themselves with peppermint and decorated their tables with it, but it came into general use in Europe as late as the 18th century. The oldest peppermint growing district in England is Mitcham in Surrey.

Peppermint water and spirit of peppermint are official preparations of the British pharmacopoeia. In flatulent colic spirit of peppermint in hot water is a good remedy. An infusion of equal quantities of peppermint and elderflowers (to which either yarrow or boneset may be added) will banish a cold or mild attack of influenza in 36 hours. Peppermint tea is also used for palpitations and insomnia as well as being a delicious drink in its own right. The bruised fresh leaves will relieve local pains and headaches. Menthol is used against rheumatic pain, neuralgia, toothache, lumbago and seasickness.

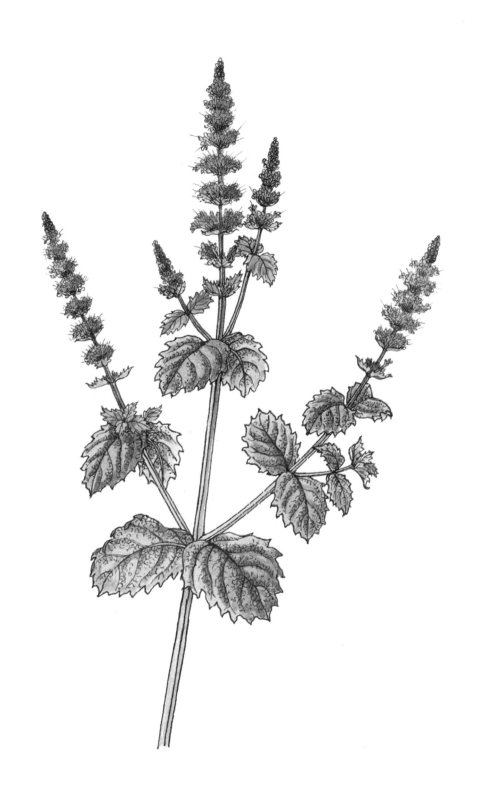

St John's Wort

Hypericum perforatum
Hyperiaceae

A pretty perennial plant in grassland and open scrub in Britain as well as all over Europe and Asia. St John's wort is cultivable in Australasia. It grows to 1 metre (3ft) and the leaves have translucent spots on them which are the oil-producing cells. The flowers are golden yellow from June to September. The English and German names are from the connection of the plant with John the Baptist.

This plant was used for healing wounds, and was hung in doors and windows to prevent the entry of evil spirits. It has been known since the days of Dioscorides and played an important role in the Middle Ages. There are many legends and superstitions attached to this plant, which traditionally flowers on the day of the summer solstice.

For chronic catarrh and throat and lung complaints an infusion is taken, and St John's wort oil (the flowers are infused in olive oil) is still a remedy for strains, sprains, cuts and bruises. 30g (1oz) of the dried herb is infused in 600ml (1 pint) of water and 1–2 tablespoons taken as a dose.

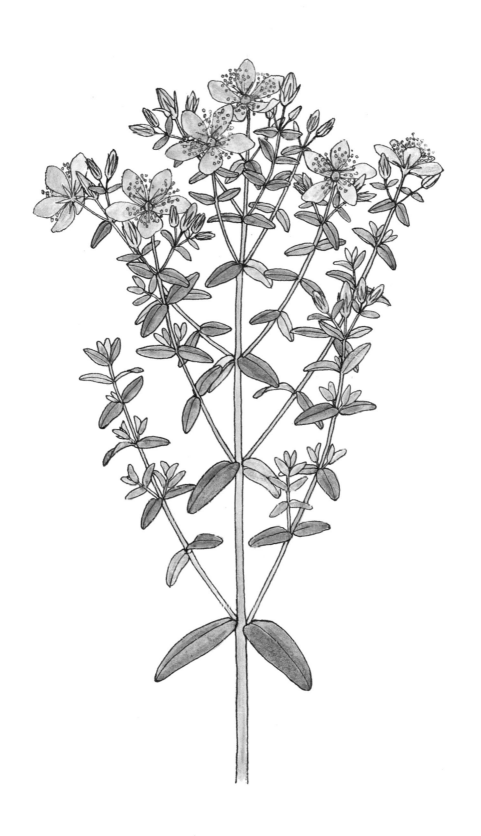

Greater Burnet Saxifrage

Pimpinella major
Umbellifereae

This plant is very like burnet saxifrage but larger in all its parts, and it has much the same medicinal properties. The root however is very acrid, and it is the leaves and seeds which are used, the seeds being carminative like those of so many of this family, notably dill and caraway. Greater burnet saxifrage is the plant illustrated, but see also burnet saxifrage below, which is more commonly found.

The older herbalists such as Pliny apparently thought a great deal of greater burnet saxifrage, although it is not held in quite such esteem these days. Aniseed is a related species of this genus which grows on the continent of Europe. The oil and resins in the dried root are effective against indigestions, and a decoction is said to remove freckles as well as being used as a gargle in cases of hoarseness.

Culpeper: 'This plant has the properties of the parsleys, but eases paines and provokes urine more effectually . . . the seed is good for cramps.'

Burnet Saxifrage

Pimpinella saxifraga
Umbellifereae

A very curious name for this plant as it is neither a burnet or a saxifrage but another member of the Umbellifers, the parsley, carrot, fennel and hogweed family. It grows throughout Europe, and the upper and lower leaves differ in size, the upper ones being fine feathery and carrot-like. Burnet saxifrage is an evergreen.

The root contains an essential oil the properties of which are antispasmodic, stomachic and diuretic. From this root is made a tincture which is given for sore throats, pharyngitis, laryngitis and bronchitis. The fresh root is antidiarrhoeic. The tincture is also prescribed in homeopathy for headaches and nose bleeding.

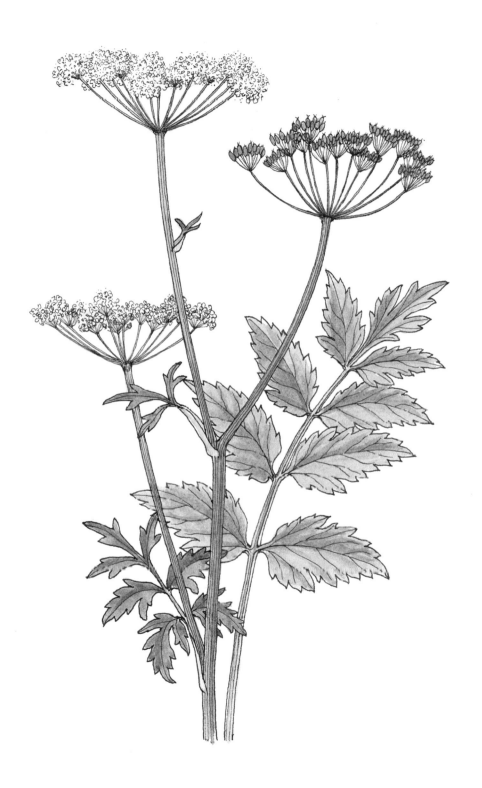

Henbane

Hyoscyamus niger
Solanaceae

A foul smelling and **extremely poisonous** annual or biennial plant growing 40–120cm (1.5–4ft) and covered with white sticky hairs. All parts of this plant contain a narcotic drug called hyoscine.

It is sedative, analgesic and spasmolytic, if the dose is increased it becomes narcotic. Henbane oil is produced from the leaves and is used for eye disorders and rheumatism. In homeopathy a tincture produced from the fresh plant is prescribed as a sedative. In some countries it is used as an aphrodisiac, and in early times it was used, very dangerously, in love potions. Dioscorides and Pliny mention it and henbane was a popular plant in sorcery. Growing in central and southern Europe and western Asia henbane belongs to the same family as the potato, tomato and deadly nightshade.

Henbane must be treated with great respect as it is poisonous in all its parts and neither drying nor boiling destroy the toxicity. Witches and sorcerers used it and it was also important in magic and diabolism for its power to throw people into convulsions.

Henbane leaves are official in all pharmacopoeias. The leaves are used as a narcotic medicine, similar in action and effect to belladonna, for relief of painful spasmodic muscle cramps, for asthma and in cases of hysteria.

Culpeper: 'All the herbs which delight most to grow in saturnine places are saturnine herbs.'

A plant to steer very clear of, henbane should only be handled by experts.

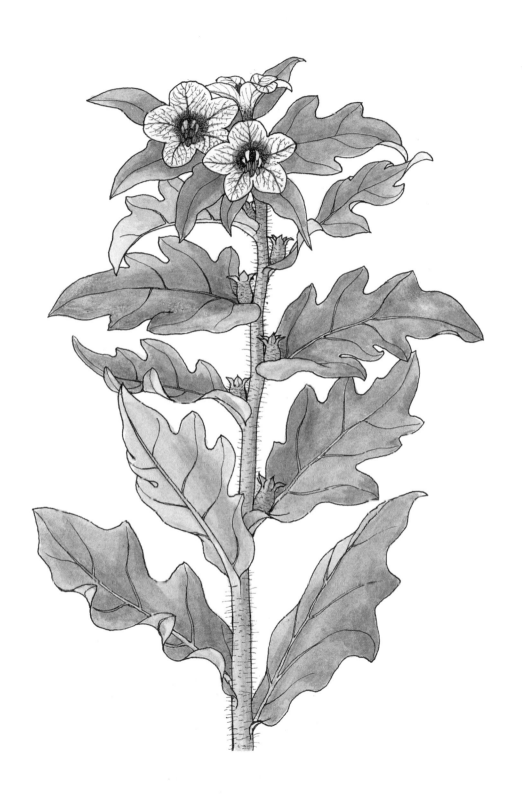

Bergamot

Monarda didyma
Rustaceae

The scarlet Monarda has become popular in gardens as the shaggy red flowers are decorative and the whole plant has a sweet fragrance. It is known in the United States of America as Oswego tea because an infusion of the leaves was widely drunk, and also as bee balm, since bees love the flowers. This ornamental plant likes a light soil and is ideally situated in a place where the flowers will get only the morning sun. It is easily propogated by cuttings or the creeping roots.

Oswego tea is a very useful tisane, it was drunk by the American Indians and the colonists used it instead of ordinary tea when boycotting British tea at the time of the Boston Tea Party. This tisane, taken hot, has a soothing and relaxing effect. Bergamot is one of the very few herbs to come from the New World to the Old, most of them going the other way. Bergamot also grows well in Australasia.

Bergamot tea drunk hot induces sleep and has a generally relaxing effect. The leaves can be added to Indian or China tea, or to wine or lemonade.

Bergamot tea: Simmer 1 teaspoon dried bergamot per cup for 10 minutes in an enamel or stainless steel saucepan. Sweeten with honey if wished.

Bergamot milk is a good nightcap: Pour 300ml (0.5 pint) boiling milk over 1 tablespoon shredded, dried leaves. Steep for at least five minutes. Strain and serve hot. Honey and lemon can be added.

The dried red flowers can also be used to make a tisane.

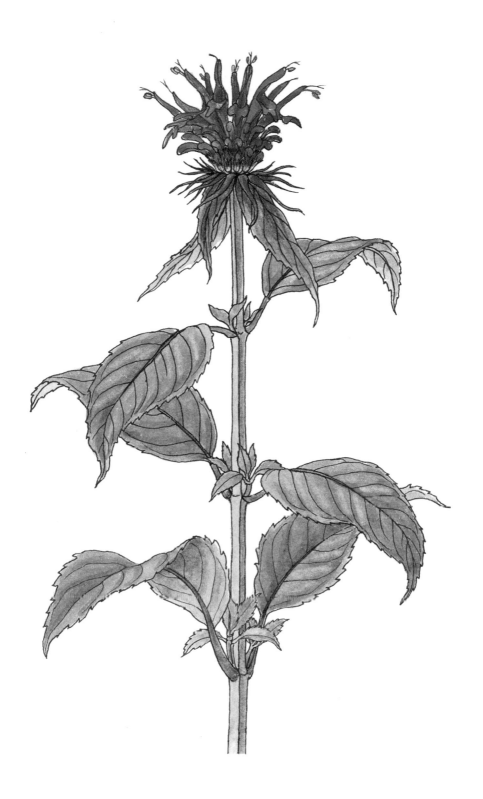

Wormwood

Artemesia absinthium
Compositeae

A perennial of the artemisia family widespread in central and southern Europe, Asia and parts of the United States, it is found infrequently in waste places in the British Isles, although wormwood is nothing like as common as its cousin mugwort. Four artemisias grow wild in Britain: common wormwood (*A. absinthium*), mugwort, sea wormwood and field wormwood. They are related to the silver-leaved garden artemisias like southernwood, and the herb tarragon. Wormwood has grooved stems and silky grey downy leaves and clusters of yellow flowers from July to August, and the entire plant is aromatic. It grows 50cm (20in) high.

Wormwood contains an essential oil and a glyocide-absinthinine which forms the bitter component. It is an excellent bitter tonic; it is antiseptic, diuretic, a vermifuge and one of the best gastric tonics used for dyspepsia and liver complaints. The liquor made from it—absinthe—affects the nervous system, and prolonged use of it leads to total degeneration, and is prohibited by law in many places. Its pharmaceutical use is much reduced but in the past it was highly prized and was much used as a tonic, against scrofula, anaemia, arthritis and as an abortive. Wormwood should only be prescribed by trained homeopaths.

Thomas Tusser (1577) mentions its use as a strewing herb, with rue, against fleas, it was also laid among the linen to keep away moths. Rue and wormwood are the bitterest herbs known.

Mességué says its concentrated bitterness contains a deadly poison. In weak doses it is an aperient similar to anise or fennel, but in strong doses it is an addictive drug. It is thus most important to keep always to the recommended dose as it is a powerful plant: exceed it and there could be serious consequences.

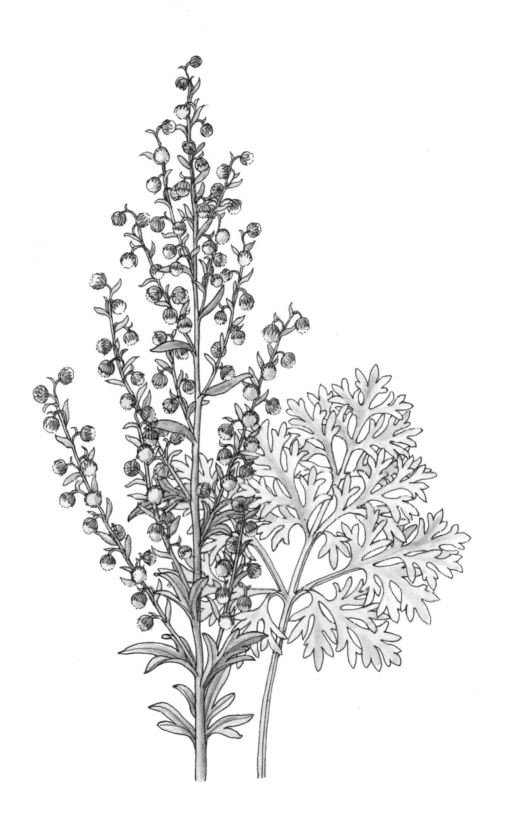

Golden Rod

Solidago vigaurea
Compositae

A common plant on dunes, in woods and heaths and moorlands, throughout Western Europe and north Asia, it grows 10–60cm (4–24in), with dentate leaves and pinicles of bright yellow flowers from July to September. Golden rod is diuretic, expectorant, anti-diarrhoeic, aromatic, stimulant, and carminative. Used externally it sooths inflammation and encourages healing. An extract, infusion or tincture can be used to treat chronic nephritis, arthritis and eczema. In homeopathy a tincture is made from the fresh flowers and used for kidney disorders.

Culpeper: 'Venus rules this herb. It is a balsamic vulnerary herb, long famous against inward hurts and bruises . . . it is a sovereign wound herb, inferior to none.'

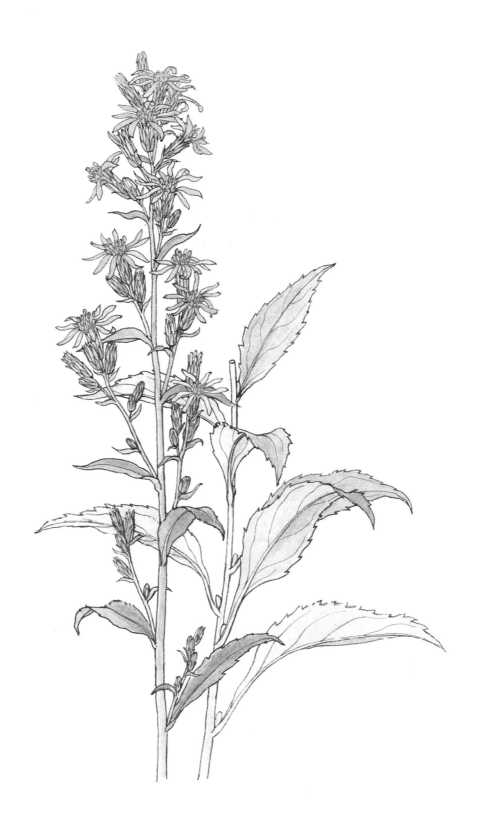

Centaury

Centaureum umbellatum
Gentianaceae

A small annual up to 30cm (1ft) high, with a single stem and clusters of pink flowers from June to August, centaury is common in dry woods and grassy places. The plant contains bitter compounds and is used in the same way as yellow gentian. It is aromatic, bitter, stomachic and tonic, acting on the liver and kidneys, and purifying the blood. It is one of the most efficacious of the wild herbs which serve as simple tonics, sharing the therapeutic virtues of yellow gentian and buck bean.

The whole herb is used, collected in July when the flowers are opening, and dried. It is given in infusion or powder form or made into an extract, and used in treating dyspepsia, for languid digestion and heartburn. 30g (1oz) of the dried herb to 600ml (1 pint) water is the infusion. When run down and suffering from loss of appetite a wineglass of this centaury tea taken 3 or 4 times daily, half an hour before meals, is of great benefit. It is also taken in the same doses for muscular rheumatism.

Culpeper: 'The herb is so safe that you cannot fail in the using of it, only give it inwardly for inward diseases, use it outwardly for outward diseases. 'Tis very wholesome but not very toothsome . . . They are under the dominion of the Sun, as appears in that their flowers open and shut as the sun either sheweth or hideth his face.' Culpeper also said centaury cleared the eyes from dimness and cured adder bites.

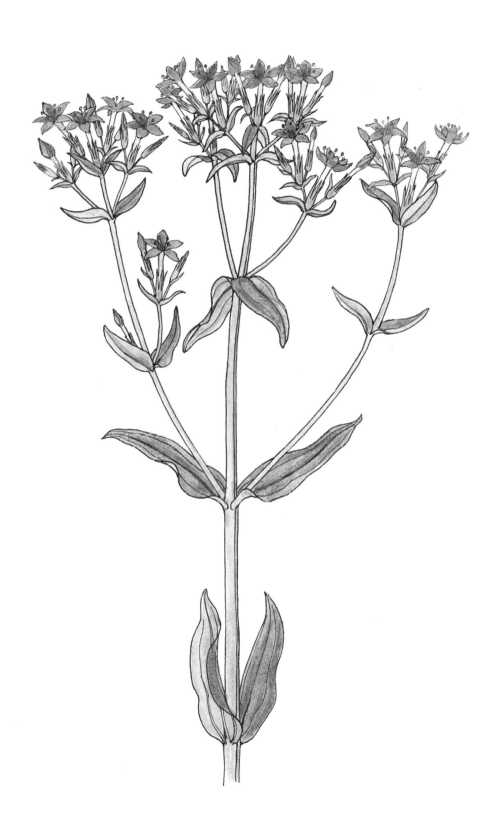

Yarrow

Milfoil
Achillea millefolium
Compositeae

Yarrow is a perennial plant with ribbed flowering stems, 30–60cm (1–2ft) high. The leaves are finely divided, hence the name milfoil, or thousand leaves, and the white or pinkish flowers are grouped in tight, flat clusters. It is common all over Europe, by roadsides and in meadows, where it flowers from June to September. It is cultivable in Australasia. The Latin name comes from Achilles who, when wounded at the siege of Troy, was told by the weeping Aphrodite to dress his wound with yarrow to ease the pain. It has always been used to ease or heal wounds, particularly wounds of war and battle, and so has other names such as woundwort and knight's milfoil. It was still used very recently in the Highlands for this purpose. Milfoil tea is drunk in the Orkney Isles to dispel melancholy.

In ancient days it was one of the herbs dedicated to the devil, and was used for divination in spells; dried yarrow stems are still used today when consulting the *I Ching*, the Chinese book of changes. It was also used as a snuff or 'old man's pepper', and put under pillows to give the sleeper a glimpse of a future wife or husband. In the 17th century it was used in salads. The capacity of the herb to stop bleeding caused it to be carried by soldiers in battle.

The whole plant is used apart from the roots, and it is diaphoretic, astringent, tonic and stimulant. Yarrow tea is a good remedy for severe colds: take 30g (1oz) dried herb to 600ml (1 pint) boiling water, drunk warm in wineglassful doses.

Mességué has used it for angina and for nervous troubles, and for women's problems at puberty and the menopause. It is a purifying agent and is used for sores, ulcers, piles and nosebleeds.

Culpeper: 'Venus governs this useful plant.' Culpeper also recommends it to be sniffed up the nose to promote sneezing, and used thus against headaches, another name for this absolutely splendid herb being 'sneezewort'.

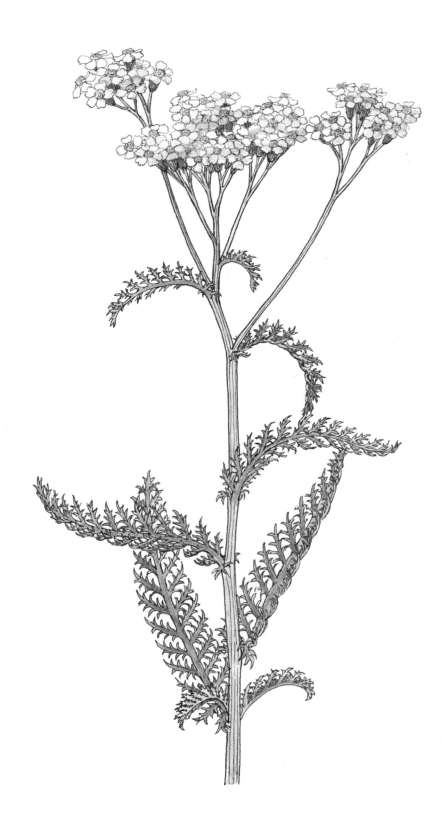

Flax

Linum usitatissimum
Linaceae

This is the cultivated flax, grown throughout Europe, and found wild on waste banks and embankments. It is a delicate annual plant 30–100cm (1–3ft) high, with bright blue flowers. It is a herb grown for its seeds, called linseed, and included in the British pharmacopoeia. It flowers in June and July.

The seeds are soothing and pain relieving as well as laxative, the oil is rich in unsaturated fatty acids. Powdered flax seeds are used in poultices, and an infusion is good for the digestive system and the urinary tract. The cultivation of flax goes back into the remote past, seeds of it have been found in Roman tombs as well as the woven cloth made from the plant—linen. The fruit is a globular capsule about the size of a pea, and contains ten seeds. The oil is obtained from the seeds, much used by painters as it forms a hard finish. Boiled oil dries more rapidly and is used to make printers' ink and by cabinet makers as a wood finish.

Medicinally linseed is employed as an addition to cough mixtures. Linseed tea is a domestic remedy for colds, taken with honey and lemon juice: 2 tablespoons of whole linseed in a jug with sliced lemon and 600ml (1 pint) of boiling water poured over. Linseed oil makes an excellent application for bruises and sprains, and 'carron oil' (first used in the Carron Iron Works) which is equal parts of linseed oil and lime water, is an embrocation for small injuries, burns and for rheumatism and gout.

Culpeper: 'Mercury owns this useful plant.'

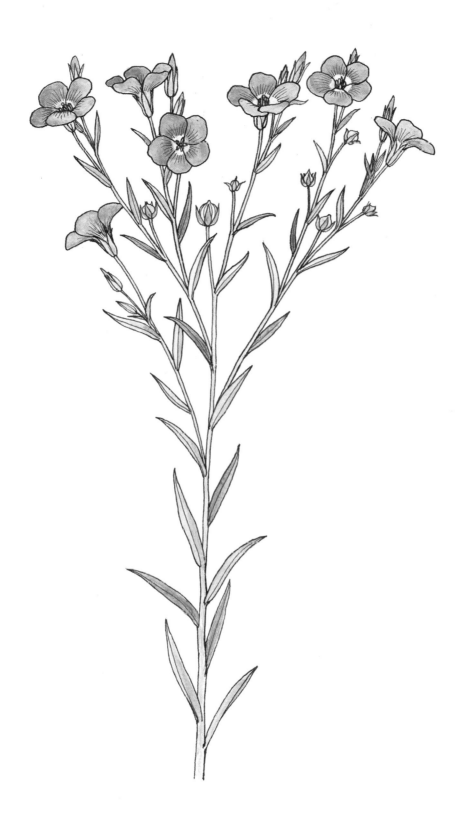

Meadowsweet

Filipendula ulmaria
Rosaceae

Meadowsweet is a perennial plant growing throughout Europe in damp fields and woods, 60–130cm (25–50in) tall with fernlike leaves and lacy tufts of creamy white flowers, very sweet smelling. This was one of the most popular strewing herbs and a favourite of Good Queen Bess. Gerard said of it: 'The leaves and flowers of Meadowsweet farre excelle all other strewing herbs for to decke up houses, to strawe in chambers, halls and banqueting houses, for the smell thereof makes the heart merrie and joyful and delighteth the senses.'

Meadowsweet, watermint and vervain were the three herbs held most sacred by the druids. The flowers were often put into wine and beer in Chaucer's time. Flowers were boiled in wine and used for ague and to cheer the heart, and the distilled flower water was used as an eye lotion.

Meadowsweet is aromatic, astringent, diuretic and sub-tonic. It is a valuable medicine in diarrhoea, particularly for children. An infusion of 30g (1oz) of the dried herb to 600ml (1 pint) of water in wineglassful doses, sweetened with honey is a good tonic. Medicinally (*Flor. Spiraeae*) is used as an infusion effective in treating rheumatism, arthritis and oedema.

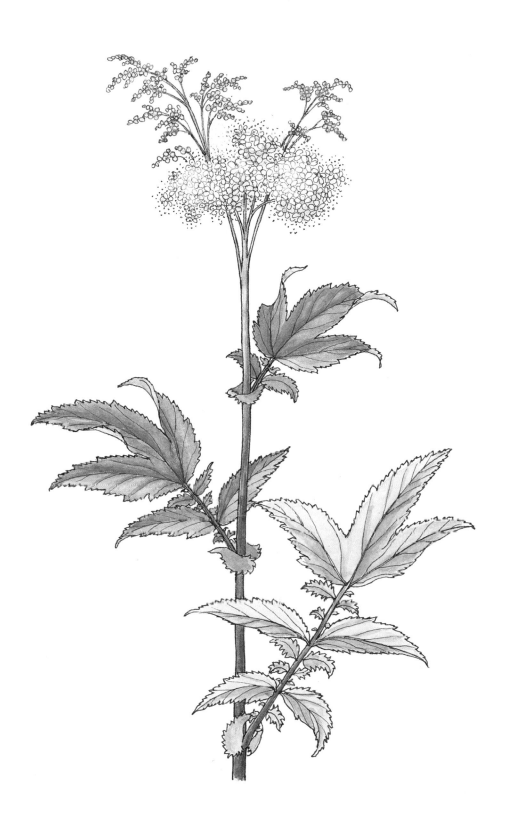

White Bryony

Bryonia dioica
Cucurbitacese

This vine-like climbing plant is the only British member of the cucumber and marrow family, just as black bryony (no relation) is the only member of the yam family. It grows all over Europe and is very common in the south of England.

It is extremely **poisonous,** as is shown in the French name, navet du diable. The flowers bloom in May and are small and greenish. The berries are pale scarlet and pea sized and hang like decorative beads on the stems when the leaves have withered, and are very toxic. It was a favourite medicine with the old herbalists, used by the Greeks and Romans, prescribed by Galen and Dioscorides, and mentioned by Gerard. There is an account of Augustus Caesar wearing a wreath of bryony to protect himself from lightning.

Culpeper: 'They are furious martial plants, the root of briony purges the belly with great violence, troubling the stomach and burning the liver, and therefore not rashly to be taken.' He goes on to say that it is good for many complaints: 'stitches in the side, palsies, cramps, convulsions.' Not surprisingly, its use as a purgative has been discontinued.

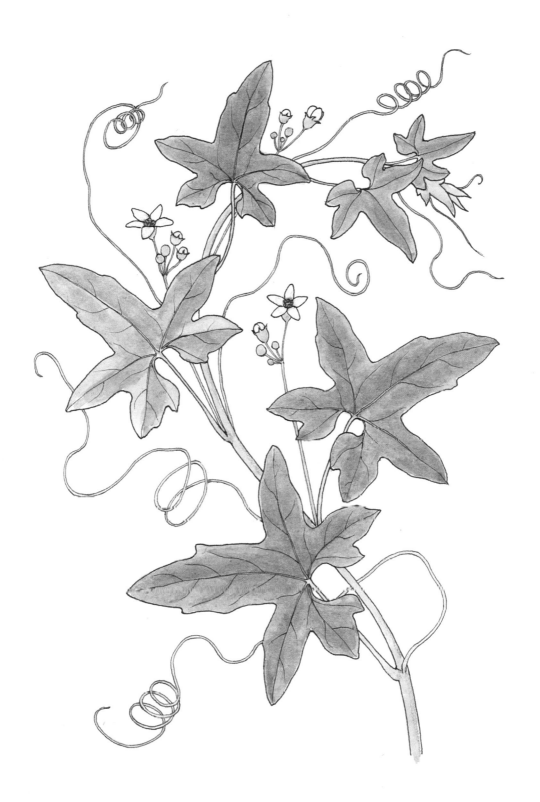

Caraway

Carum carvi
Umbelliferae

Common in Europe and north Asia, and cultivable in Australia, caraway is not often found in the wild in England, but grows well in gardens as a herb plant. It has large umbels of white flowers from May to July, finely divided leaves and is a pretty biennial. It is a member of the group of aromatic umbelliferous plants with carminative or soothing characteristics like dill, fennel, cumin and anise. It is usually grown for the flavouring properties of its seeds, much used in cooking, confectionery and liqueurs such as kümmel. As an infusion it is used medicinally to treat rheumatism and pleurisy.

Caraway was known in Roman times and Dioscorides advised pale faced girls to take it. In *Henry IV* Justice Shallow invites Falstaff to a 'pippin and a dish of caraways'. The seeds were used a great deal with baked fruit and put into bread and cakes. Caraway seed cake was eaten during celebrations at the end of wheat sowing, and in Germany the seeds are used much more than in Britain to flavour bread, cheese, cabbage dishes and soups. It was once a popular ingredient in love potions to prevent the lovers proving fickle. Both the fruit (seeds) and the oil are aromatic, stimulant and carminative. Caraway water is considered a useful remedy for flatulence, indigestion and colic.

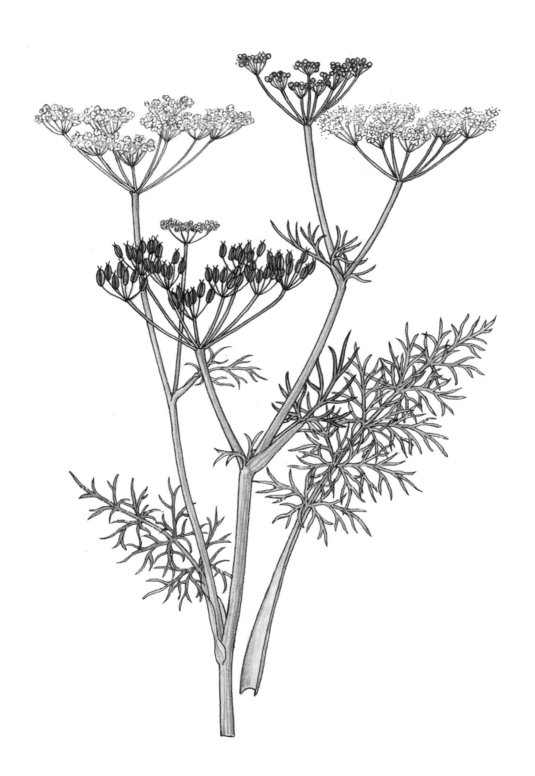

Sage

Salvia officinalis
Labiatae

Sage is a small shrub with wrinkled grey aromatic leaves and spikes of violet flowers, growing in southern Europe and the Mediterranean countries, and grown in Britain for centuries in kitchen and herb gardens. Gerard mentioned it as being well known in 1597 and grew many varieties in his garden at Holborn. The use of sage in the kitchen needs no description as it has from time immemorial been associated with fatty foods such as pork and goose, and it is an indispensible ingredient in stuffings.

Sage has also long been used as a tisane or tea, the Chinese at one time preferring sage tea to their own tea, and bartering for it with the Dutch traders. The leaves are eaten in country districts with bread and butter, particularly in May, hence the old rhyme: 'He who would live for aye, Must eat of Sage in May.' Garden sage needs a warm, rather dry border, but will grow almost anywhere. It is a hardy plant, propogated every 3 or 4 years by rooting cuttings.

The medical action is stimulant, astringent, tonic and carminative. The infusion known as sage tea is simply made by pouring 600ml (1 pint) of boiling water onto 30g (1oz) of dried sage, and half a teacupful is taken when required. It is cooling in fevers and is a cleanser and purifier of the blood, and it is also a refreshing drink. Another method is to infuse 15g (0.5oz) of fresh sage leaves, 30g (1oz) sugar and the juice of a lemon for half an hour. Both these stimulant tonics are useful for gargles and sore throats.

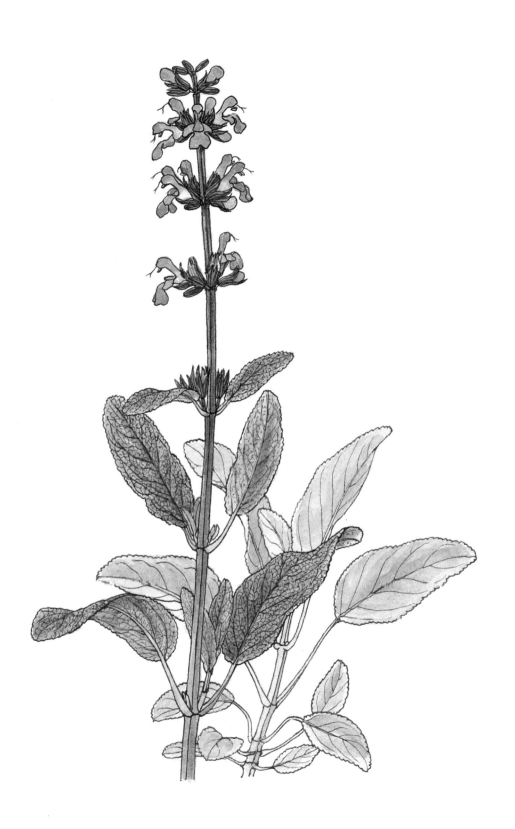

Elder

Sambucus niger
Caprifoliaceae

Elder grows in small trees, common on waysides in Europe, west Asia and north America, with deciduous leaves and flat clusters of creamy white, sweet smelling flowers in June and July. The flowers are followed by black fruits.

The elder has many traditions associated with it. The tree was planted by houses to keep away witches, and it was considered very bad luck to cut down an elder tree in the hedgerow or to burn its wood. In Norse countries the tree was under the protection of a dryad called Hylde-Moer, the elder mother, and if a tree was cut down and furniture made from the wood Hylde-Moer would follow and haunt the transgressors. Indeed many countries have a tradition of asking permission of the spirit of the tree before cutting elder, and there is an old belief that if you stand under an elder tree on Midsummer Eve you see the King of Fairyland and all his train go by. In spite of all this elder wood was used for butchers' skewers, and small turned articles like weaving needles, combs and small toys.

Both the flowers and the berries were, and are, made into wine, and the berries, rich in vitamin C, are made into a winter cordial and cold cure. Elder flowers, fresh or dried, are the basis for many tisanes which are both healthy and sleep inducing. They keep their sweet scent of summer. John Evelyn said: 'If the medicinal properties of its leaves, bark and berries were fully known, I cannot tell what our countryman could ail for which he might not fetch a remedy from every hedge, either for sickness or wounds.'

Elderflower water (*Aqua Sambuci*) is used as a base for mixing medicines but chiefly as a vehicle for eye and skin lotions; it is mildly astringent and stimulant. Elderflower tea is an old-fashioned remedy for colds and chills and a good tonic medicine to be taken every morning before breakfast for some weeks. Elderberries are used for wine, and as additions to jams and as a cordial. Hot elderberry wine with cinnamon is a good remedy for colds and asthma.

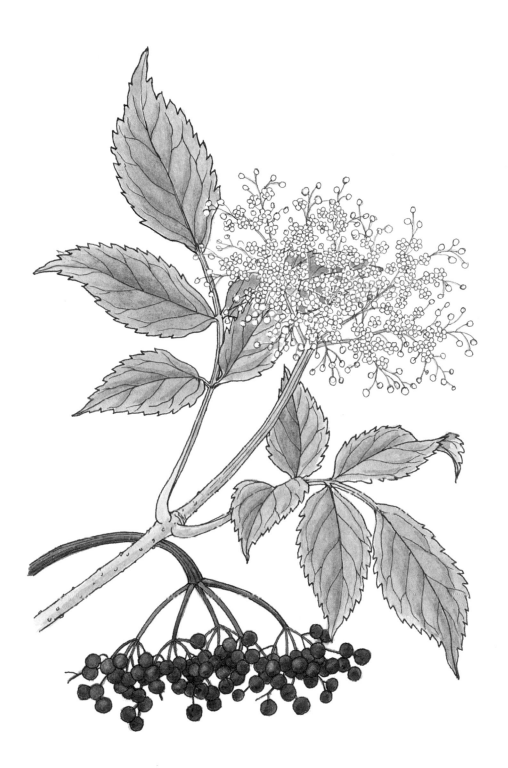

Restharrow

Ononis spinosa
Leguminosae

Restharrow is a fairly common weed on sandy and chalky soils throughout Europe, it is a rough spiny perennial plant with a tough creeping stem and purple-red pea-like flowers from July to September. The young shoots were used as a vegetable in ancient times, and in medieval days restharrow was used medicinally for stone in the bladder and to subdue delerium. The root (*Radix Ononidis*) contains an essential oil which is a diuretic. An infusion of flowers and roots is used by herbalists for disorders of the urinary tract.

Culpeper: 'It is under the dominion of Mars. It is excellent to provoke urine.'

Gerard: 'The root is long and runneth far abroad, very tough, and hard to be torn to pieces with the plough, insomuch that the oxen can hardly passe forward, but are constrained to stand still; whereupon it was called Res-Plough or Rest-Harrow!' Gerard also says that: 'The tender sprigs or crops of this shrub before the thorns come forth, are preserved in pickle, and be very pleasant sauce to be eaten with meat as a sallad.'

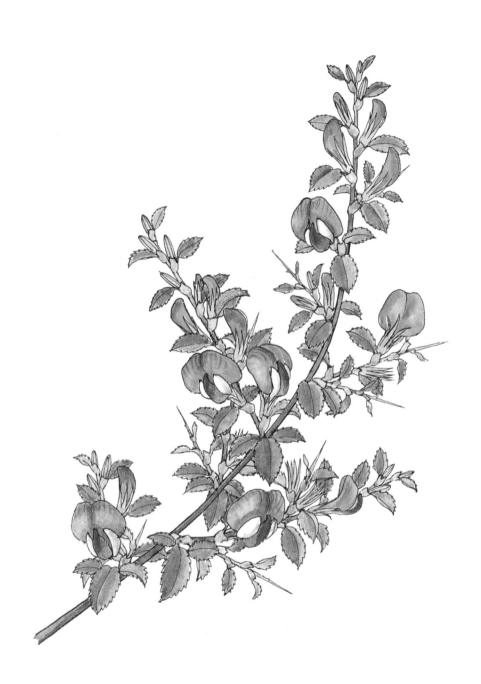

Hop

Humulus lupulus
Cannabaceae

The hop is a well known twining and climbing perennial growing in damp woodlands and hedgerows in Europe, Asia and North America, cultivable in Australasia, and common in Britain in Kent and Worcestershire for use in brewing. Hops were cultivated by the Romans, but were not grown in England until the 16th century. The female flowers are small, green, cone shaped catkins, which contain resins and bitter aromatic substances some of which are mildly narcotic. Before the 16th century in England ale was brewed from fermented malt or a mixture of malt and honey, and flavoured with marjoram, wormwood, yarrow or buck bean. Henry VIII forbade brewers to put hops into ale as was done in Holland: 'The hop being a wicked weed that would spoil the taste of the drink and endanger the people.' Hops were at first thought to engender melancholy.

John Evelyn (1670) wrote that: 'Hops transmuted our wholesome ale into beer which doubtless alters its constitution. This one ingredient, by some suspected not unworthily, preserves the drink indeed, but repays the pleasure in tormenting diseases and a shorter life.'

Medicinally hops have tonic, nervine, diuretic and anodyne properties. They improve the appetite and promote sleep. The official preparations are an infusion and a tincture. Both are considered sedative. An infusion of 15g (0.5oz) hops to 600ml (1 pint) water is the quantity for ordinary use. An infusion of the leaves, flowers and stalks taken by the wineglassful 2 or 3 times a day in the early spring is good for sluggish livers.

Industrially the hop is used as an aromatic bitter. The male flowers and young shoots are eaten in most hop-growing areas as a vegetable (*jets d'houblon*) with butter and cream, or parboiled and dressed with oil and lemon juice.

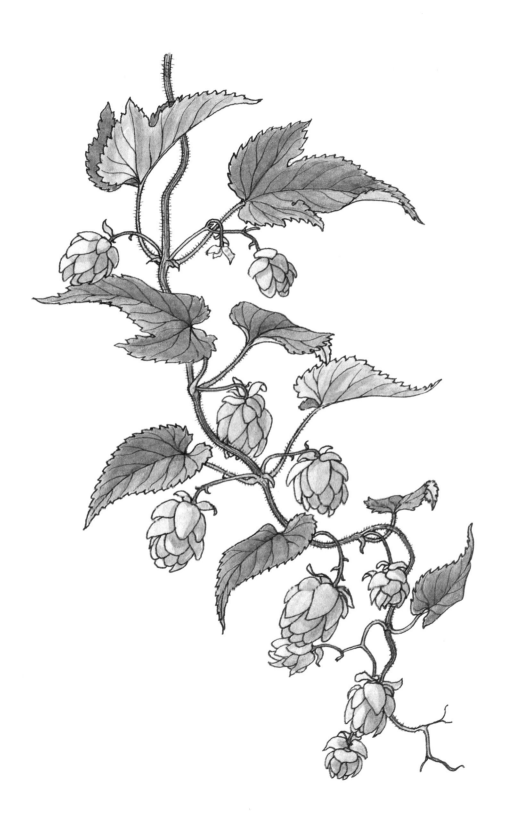

Valerian

Valeriana officinalis
Valerianaceae

Valerian is found all over Europe and is common in England in marshy thickets and on the edges of ditches and streams. The plant grows 30–60cm (1–2ft) and has feathery leaves and small, pale pink corymbs of flowers from June to August. These have a strange, almost unpleasant smell. The part used in medicine is the rhizome with the roots which produce an essential oil.

Valerian is a tranquilliser, antispasmodic and stomachic. The drug allays pain and promotes sleep, and it has none of the side or after effects produced by narcotics. It is used for nervous disorders, hysteria, neurasthenia, migraines and digestive troubles. It is wise to follow a herbalist's advice.

Culpeper: 'It is under the influence of Mercury and therefore has a warming facility.' He recommends the root boiled with liquorice, raisins and aniseed for the cough.

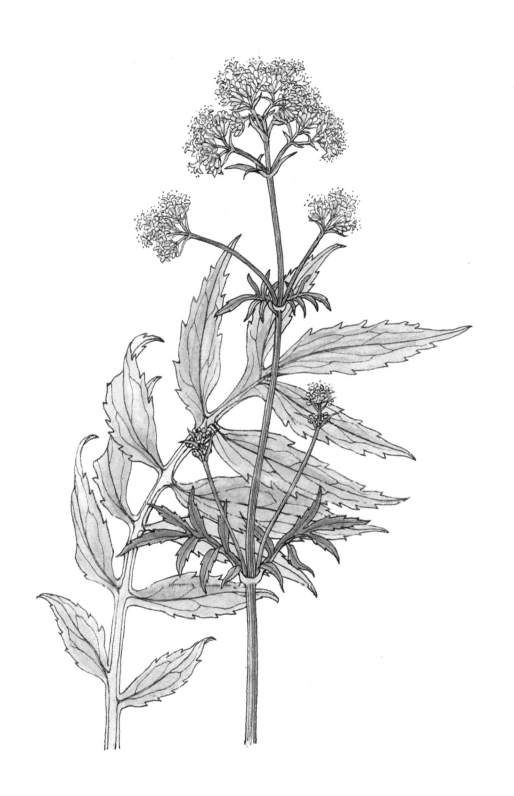

Yellow Gentian

Gentiana lutea
Gentianaceae

The yellow gentian is a native of the Alps, Carpathians and Balkan mountains, and grows in the Pyrenees, the Jura, the Vosges, the Auvergne and the Black Forest. In Great Britain it is only grown as a garden plant. All gentians are remarkable for the intensely bitter properties in their roots and every part of the plant, and because of this they are valuable as tonic medicines. Before the introduction of hops, gentian was used to make beer bitter and tonic, and it is used to make the bitter aperitifs such as suze in France.

Like all bitter plants gentian acts as a tonic for the whole digestive system. The root is used as a decoction, as an extract (*Extr. Gentianae*) or as a tincture (*Tinct. Gentianae*). The plant has been used in this way since ancient times, for Pliny and Dioscorides both mention it. It is useful in cases of exhaustion from chronic disease and in all cases of chronic debility, weakness of the digestion and loss of appetite. It has been used for anorexia nervosa. It is one of the best tonic strengtheners of the system. A tincture made with 30g (1oz) of the root, 30g (1oz) dried orange peel and 15g (0.5oz) bruised cardamom seeds in a quart of brandy is an excellent tonic, restoring appetite and promoting digestion.

Mességué: 1–3 pinches of the powder with honey as a tonic once a day for a week; he warns that the recommended dose must not be exceeded as this can cause vomiting if taken in strong doses.

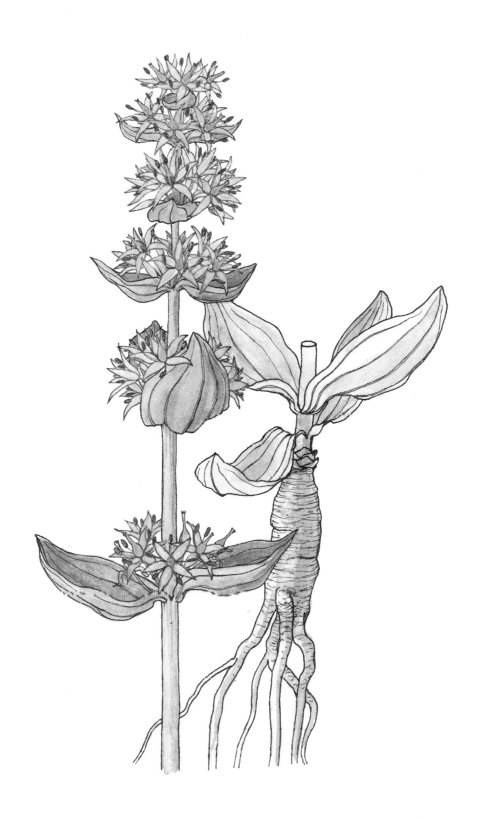

Blackberry

Bramble
Rubus fruiticosus
Roseaceae

The bramble, growing in every English hedgerow, is also found all over the world and hardly needs description. The prickly stems creep or climb and the blossoms as well as the ripe and unripe fruit may all be seen at the same time on the bushes. It is an old medicinal plant and was used because of its potency as a charm for various disorders.

An infusion made from the leaves is used in cases of internal haemorrhage, dysentry and diarrhoea (30g/1oz dried leaves infused in 600ml/1 pint boiling water, taken cold a teacupful at a time). A decoction of the leaves is used as a gargle for sore throats, pharyngitis and gingivitis. A syrup made from the fruits is particularly good for children.

Culpeper: 'It is a plant of Venus in Aries. If any ask the reason why Venus is so prickly? Tell them it is because she is in the house of Mars.'

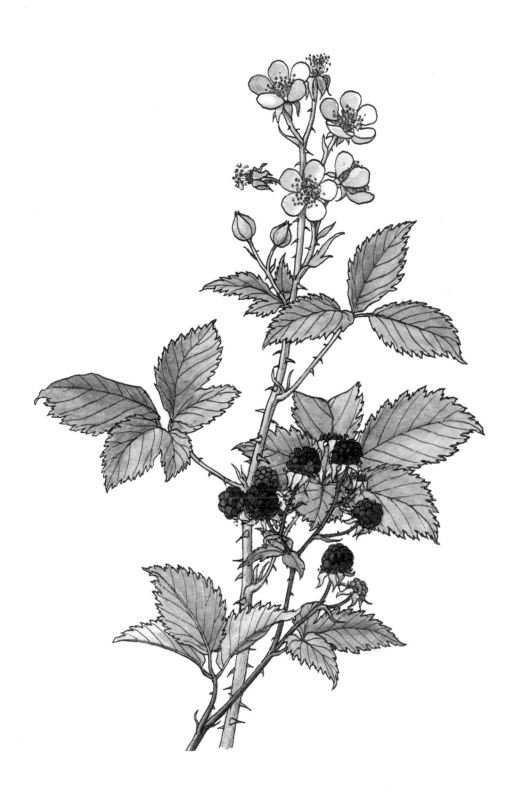

Willow

Salix purpurea
Salicaceae

Willow is a common tree found in damp woods and by rivers. The trees grow with erect branches and silvery white foliage. The bark and leaves contain glycosides and tannin. Willow is tonic, febrifuge and anti-rheumatismal, and its febrifuge properties were known in ancient Greece. It has deen used in dyspepsia, and in convalescence from acute disorders and diseases, and in chronic diarrhoea and dysentry where its tonic and astringent combination makes it very useful.

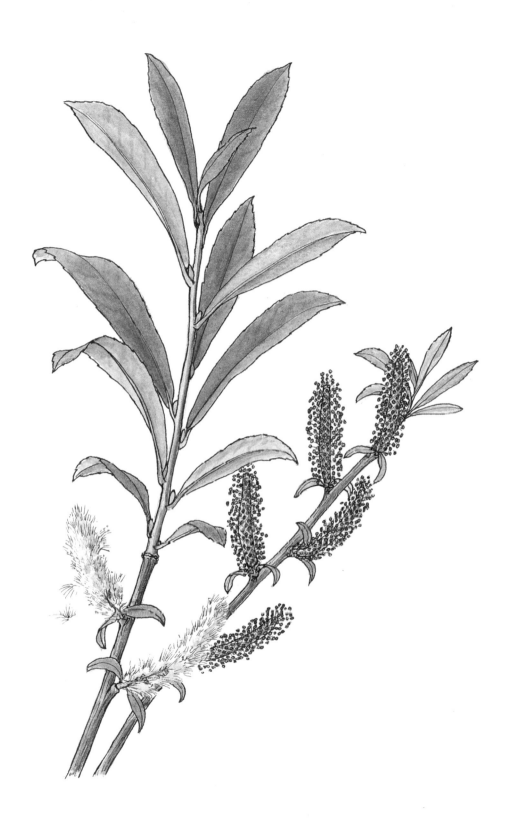

Wild Thyme

Thymus serpyllum
Labiateae

A widespread plant all over Europe, common on banks, heaths and dry grassy places in the British Isles. It is a low growing, sweet-smelling perennial with small oval leaves and tiny pink flowers from July to August.

It grows equally well as garden thyme in borders, rockeries or on walls. The plant produces an essential oil (*Ol. Serpylli*), and is a bitter aromatic, tonic, expectorant, and antispasmodic as well as a disenfectant. Wild thyme is an ingredient in many aromatic tisanes; in homeopathy it is used as an infusion, and it calms and sooths coughing.

Francis Bacon produced a plan for the perfect garden where, among other things, alleys should be planted with fragrant plants: 'Burnet, Wild Thyme and Water Mints, which perfume the air most delightfully being trodden on and crushed.' The herb denotes a pure atmosphere where it grows wild, and was believed to enliven the spirits with its fragrance. The Romans gave thyme as a remedy to melancholy persons. Bees are fond of thyme flowers, and Titania in *Midsummer Night's Dream* lived by a bank 'whereon the wild thyme blows'.

For an infusion take 30g (1oz) of the dried herb to 600ml (1 pint) boiling water, which can be sweetened with sugar or honey and is used for chest maladies and for weak digestion, being a good remedy for flatulence.

Culpeper: 'The whole plant is fragrant, and yields an essential oil that is very heating. An infusion of the leaves relieves headache occasioned by inebriation. It is under Venus and is excellent for nervous disorders. A strong infusion, drunk as a tea, is pleasant, and a very effectual remedy for headache, giddiness and other disorders of that kind, and a certain remedy for that troublesome complaint, the Night Mare.'

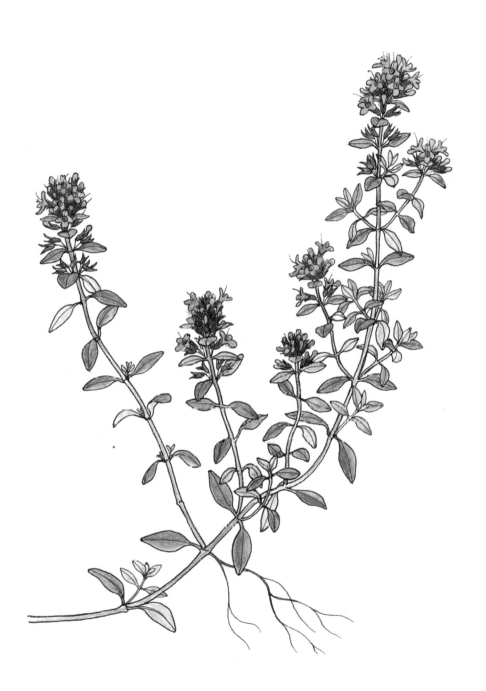

Horse Chestnut

Aesculus hippocastanium
Hippocastanaceae

Horse chestnut is a well-known and loved tree, growing up to 30 metres (90ft) with large palmate leaves, 'sticky' buds in winter, candles of white or pink flowers in May, and 'conkers', large brown shining seeds in a prickly case, in autumn. The chestnut comes from northern and central Asia and was introduced into Great Britain about the middle of the 16th century.

The bark and the fruit are used medicinally. The bark has tonic, narcotic and febrifuge properties and is used in intermittent fevers, and as an external application to ulcers. The fruits have been used in the treatment of rheumatism, neuralgia and for haemorrhoides (*Fruct. hippocastanii*). The fluid extract from the fruits is an antiphlogistic and diuretic in cases of venous (vein) origin—varicose veins and haemorrhoides. It increases the rate of blood circulation and is used in cases of gastritis, enteritis and prostate malfunction. Horse chestnut should only be taken by prescription.

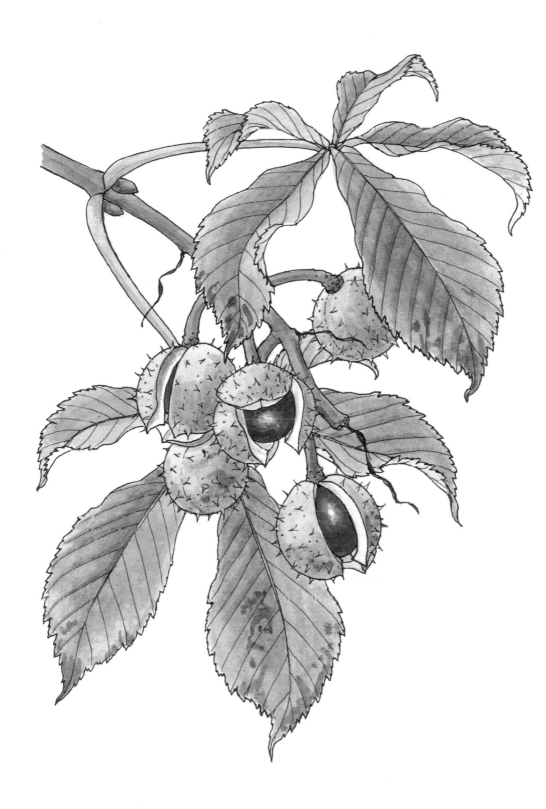

Great Mullein

Verbascum thapsus
Scrophulariaceae

A woolly biennial plant, growing 120cm (4ft) or more tall with a rosette of leaves the first year from which the flower spike grows in the second year. It is common on dry soils in sunny places. The almost stalkless flowers are yellow and open in a higgledy-piggledy cluster around the spike. The down on the leaves and stems burns well when dry and was, before the introduction of cotton, used for lamp wicks. Both in Asia and Europe mulleins were considered safeguards against evil spirits and magic; Ulysees took a plant with him to help protect him from the wiles of Circe.

The leaves and flowers are the parts used in medicine. Fresh mullein leaves are also used for the purposes of making a homeo-pathic tincture. The properties are soothing and expectorant. The flowers (*Flor. Verbasci*) are official, they can be used as a decoction or an infusion. In early medicine the roots were used.

Mességué says: 'The golden flowers soften the tissues and prepare them for healing.' The flowers are marvellous for all irrita-tions of the respiratory system. They are good for chills, tonsillitis, bronchitis, pneumonia, pulmonary congestion and pleurisy. The soothing virtues of the mullein make the plant a good treatment for asthma, nervousness, anxiety, palpitations, stomach cramp and neuralgia. The flowers are gathered and dried quickly and stored.

For an infusion of mullein flowers take half a handful of fresh or dried flowers to a litre of water, strain the infusion in order to remove the stamens. Drink 3 or 4 cups a day.

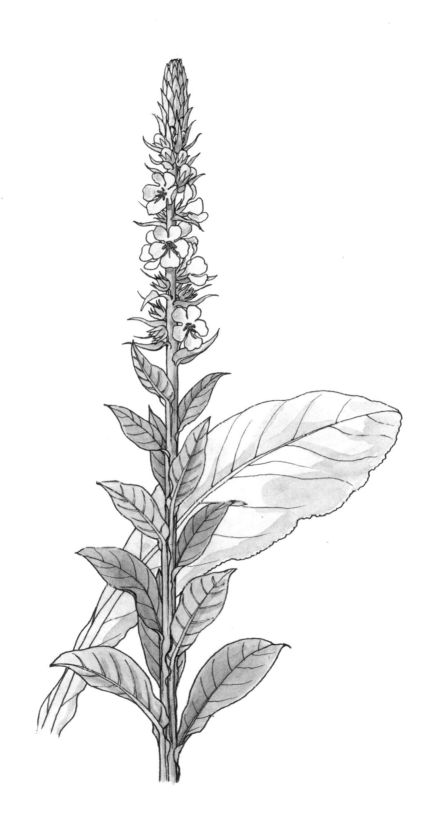

Passion Flower

Passiflora incarnata
Passifloraceae

The passion flower gets its name from the resemblance of the corona in the centre of the flower to the crown of thorns. Its original habitat is South America. The blue passion flower, *P. cerulea*, is hardy in southern districts of Great Britain and is grown as a decorative wall climber. It was introduced into England from Brazil in 1699. It has a perennial root and herbaceous shoots. The leaves are finely serated and the extraordinary fringed flowers are tinged with purple.

The active principle seems to be similar to morphine. The dried leaves are used. The drug is a depressant, official in homeopathic medicine and used with bromides. It has narcotic properties and is sometimes prescribed in cases of diarrhoea, dysentry, neuralgia, sleeplessness and dysmenorrhoea. Many of this family of plants are grown for their edible fruits.

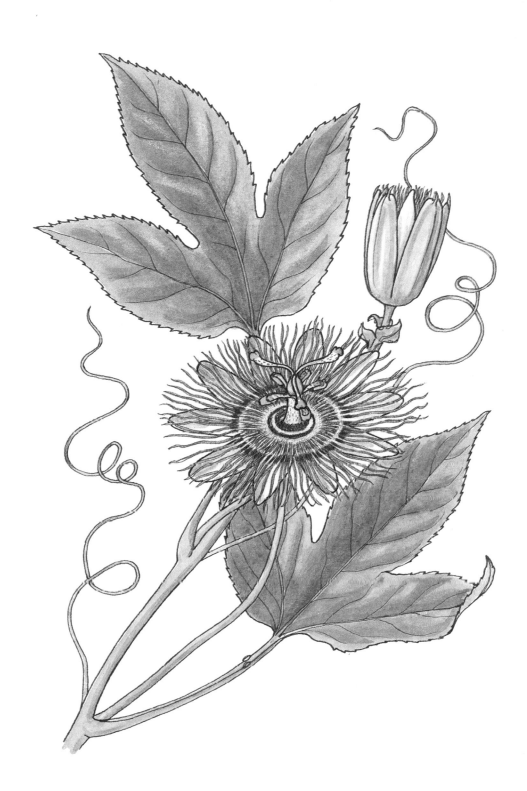

Bilberry

Whortleberry, Blueberry, Huckleberry
Vaccinum myrtillus
Vacciniaceae

Bilberries are very common, low, deciduous shrubs, widespread throughout Europe on acid soils, moorlands, peat bogs and coniferous forests. The bushes are 25–50cm (10–20in) high with oval dentate leaves, bell-shaped greenish-pink flowers and blue-black berries.

The fruit and leaves are used, the berries are an official remedy (*Fruct. Myrtilli*). They have a high nutritive value and are eaten raw or as jams and syrups. The leaves are used in the form of a decoction. The collecting season is from June to August.

Owing to its rich juice the bilberry can be used with the smallest quantities of sugar in making jam—250g (½lb) of sugar to 500g (1lb) of berries if the jam is to be eaten soon. The fruits are astringent and are valuable in the treatment of diarrhoea and dysentry in the form of a syrup. The leaves contain a substance which lowers the blood sugar level, and a tea made with them was sometimes used for diabetes.

Culpeper: 'They are under the dominion of Jupiter. It is a pity that they are used no more in physic than they are . . . They do somewhat bind the belly and stay the vomitings and loathings.'

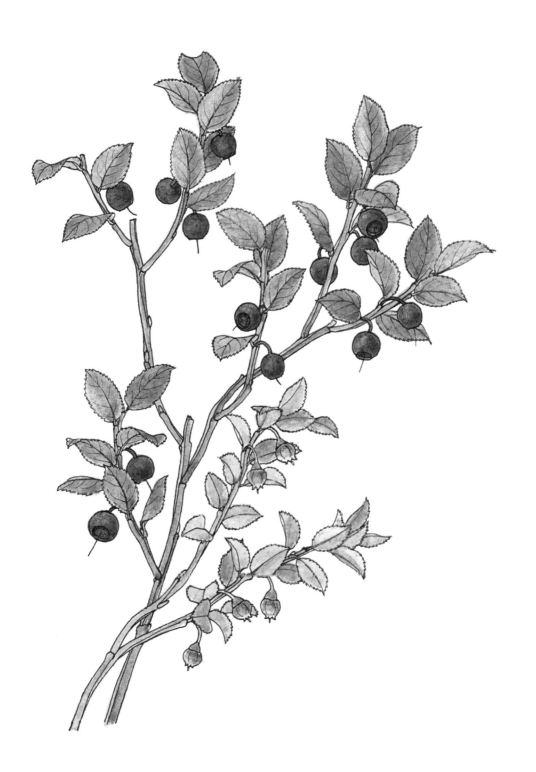

Bearberry

Arctostaphylos Uva-ursi
Ericaceae

The bearberry is an evergreen plant fairly widespread in mountain regions, with untoothed leaves which turn red in winter; the flowers are small, pink and white, and the fruits are red and shiny. It is related to the arbutus. The leaves (*Folia uvae ursi*) are used in medicines for kidney troubles, and in homeopathy a tincture of the fresh leaves is used to treat cystitis, pyelitis and gravel.

There are records that this plant was used in the 13th century, and it was being recommended in 1763. The usual form of medicine is an infusion which has a soothing as well as an astringent effect and marked diuretic action. It is of value in diseases of the bladder and kidneys. The leaves are so full of tannin that they have been used for tanning leather in Sweden and Russia. The berries are only eaten by grouse.

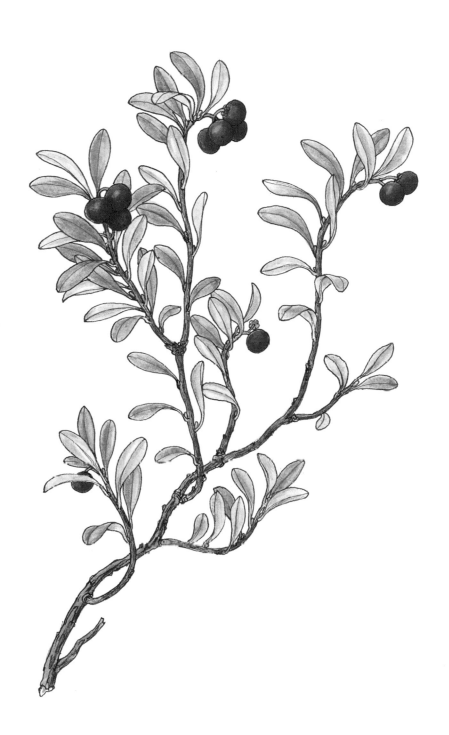

Artichoke

Cynara scolymus
Compositae

A beautiful vegetable plant grown in the Mediterranean and central Europe as a food plant, also growing well in Brittany and in Great Britain. It grows up to 1.5 metres (5ft) high and has grey-green decorative pinnate leaves, and huge purple thistle-like flowers in July and August. The flower buds are the edible parts of the plant; the leaves, stems and root contain a bitter, aromatic and chrystalline substance called cynarine. This has a strong choleretic and diuretic action and is effective against arteriosclerosis and diabetes. It is choleretic in cases of liver malfunctions, jaundice and dyspepsia, or may be given as a diuretic in post-operative anaemia, also to treat some skin disorders.

Mességué says that artichoke is so good for the circulation that it prevents many of the illnesses that are caused by cholesterol —hardening of the arteries, angina and heart disorders and attacks. In his view this plant is the best preventative medicine for people in their fifties.

Infusions and decoctions of the leaves and roots are taken, usually with honey because they are so bitter. Put half a handful of 'either leaves or roots, or equal quantities of both, into a litre of water, and take 3 cupfuls a day before meals.

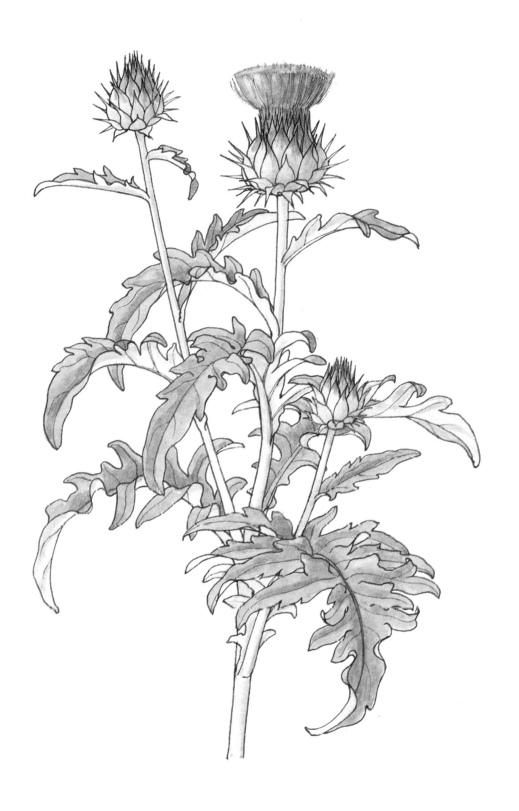

Male Fern

Aspidium filix-mas
Polypodiaceae

The male fern is one of the commonest and hardiest British ferns, and, after the bracken, the species most frequently met with in woods and moist banks and hedgerows. In sheltered places it will remain green all the winter. It is found all over Europe, temperate Asia, north India, Africa, temperate parts of the USA and in the Andes. It grows up to 120cm (4ft) in height with wide, spreading, lance-shaped fronds producing spores from June to September.

The pulverised rhizome (*Rhiz. Filicis*) and an extract of the rhizome (*Extr. Filicis*) are used as vermifuges. The male fern is **toxic** and antihelminthic. The doses must be small and accompanied by a saline purgative to prevent poisoning. It is essential to evacuate the drug within two hours of taking it. In homeopathy a tincture is used to treat septic wounds, ulcers, and varicose veins. In herbalism a decoction is made for the same purposes. The male fern was known in ancient Greece in the times of Theophrastus and Dioscorides as a valuable vermifuge.

Gerard: 'The roots of the Male Fern, being taken in the weight of half an ounce, driveth forth long, flat worms, as Dioscorides writeth, being drunke in mede or honied water, and more effectually if it be given with two scruples or two third parts of a dram of scammonie, or of black Hellebore; they that will use it must first eat garlic.'

At present the male fern seems most widely used for expelling tapeworms, mainly by vets.

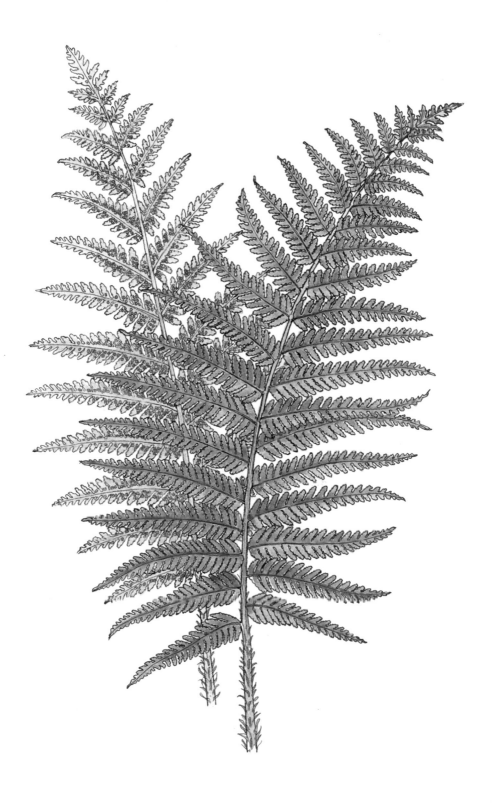

Juniper

Juniperus communis
Cupressaceae

Juniper is an evergreen shrub or small tree with needle-like leaves, growing all over the northern hemisphere; the 'berries' are really female cones, turning blueish black in the autumn of their third year. Junipers like dry, rocky soils, moorland, woodland clearings, and are common where bands of limestone appear. The strong, aromatic scent emanates from all parts of the shrub and the berries are slightly bitter-sweet, fragrant and spicy. They stimulate the appetite, are disinfectant and antibiotic, and they stimulate the function of the kidneys. Their preserving qualities are used in marinades for game, especially venison.

The berries are used for the production of the volatile oil which is an important ingredient of Geneva or Hollands Gin, and also to flavour food (there is a recipe in which pork is made to taste like wild boar by the use of juniper berries).

The oil and the bitter compound contained in the berries make them medicinally diuretic, a stomachic tonic and carminative. Juniper has a beneficial effect on the appetite and digestion. An infusion of the berries is used as a disinfectant of the urinary tract. Used externally a tincture of the branches is the treatment for a number of diseases. This plant should be avoided by people with kidney inflammation.

Culpeper: 'The berries are hot in the third degree, and dry in the first, being counter-poison, and a resister of the pestilence, and excellent against the bites of venemous beasts.'

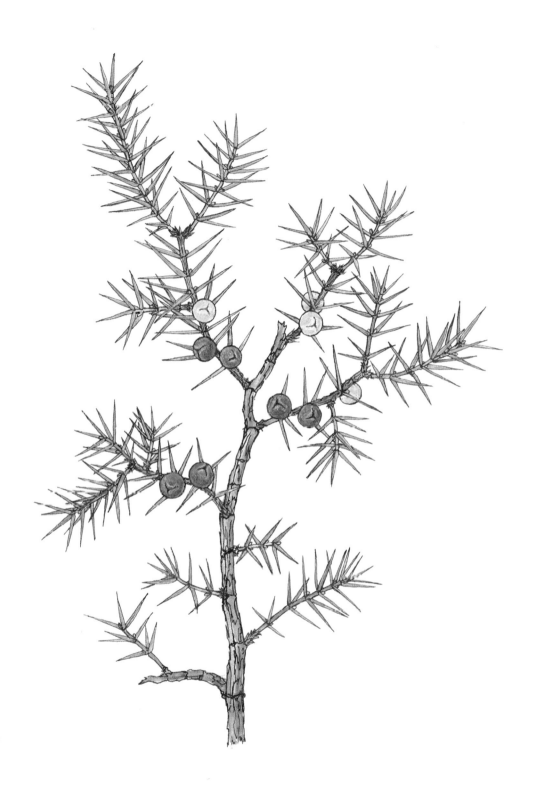

Mistletoe

Viscum album
Loranthaceae

The well-known Christmas mistletoe is an evergreen parasite, getting most of its nourishment from the trees on which it grows and thus weakening them. The stiff-branched bushes hang in the branches of trees, particularly apple, poplar and ash. The sticky white berries attract birds in winter, and it is on their beaks that they are carried from tree to tree and take root. Thrushes are the birds which love the berries most—hence the missel thrush. Mistletoe is found throughout Europe, is always produced by seed and it cannot be cultivated in the earth. In Brittany where it grows in profusion the plant is called herbe de la croix.

Mistletoe was held in great esteem by the druids who made it a sacred plant, cutting it ceremoniously from the tree with a golden knife, always at a particular age of the moon at the beginning of the year. The mistletoe was held to protect its possessor from evil, and the entrance of a new year was announced by carrying bunches of mistletoe from house to house. Possibly our Christmas 'kissing bunches' are a survival of this custom.

The whole plant is used medicinally, the preparations being usually a fluid extract and the powdered leaves. It is nervine, antispasmodic, tonic and narcotic. It has a reputation for curing the 'falling sickness'—epilepsy, and other convulsive nervous disorders. The effect is to lessen the nervous action and stop spasms. In large quantities the plant is **poisonous affecting the heart,** and children have been given convulsions by eating the berries. It has been considered a cure for epilepsy since ancient times, and as a tonic in nervous disorders, the specific herb for St Vitus's dance, and employed in cases of convulsions, delerium, hysteria and many other complaints.

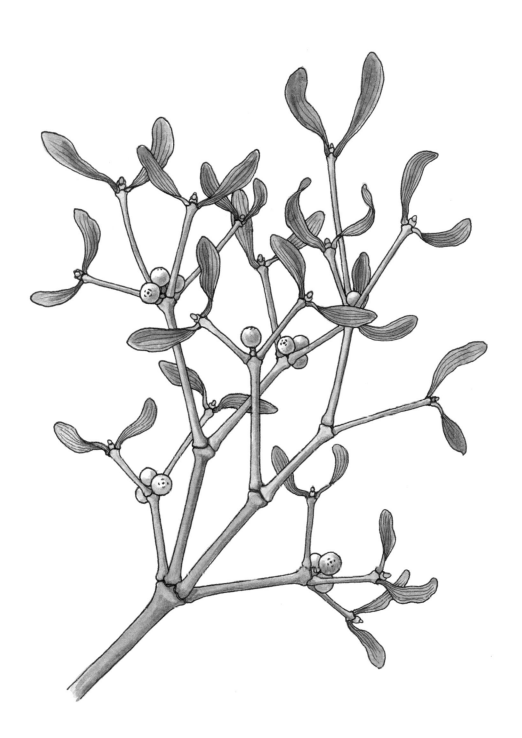

Infusions, teas and mixtures

One way to make use of the health giving properties of herbs, as well as improving food with their unique flavours, is in cooking. The other simple way is to make a herb infusion or tea. Infusions can be made with either boiling, warm or cold water according to the herb. Teas or tisanes are wholesome and health-giving drinks, some of them have a therapeutic value and some are cosmetic or may be used as bath preparations.

These teas are delicate in taste and the herbs used must be perfectly fresh or carefully dried so that the flavour is not impaired. It is a simple matter to make them but there are certain pitfalls, as many can be ruined by being steeped too long in the water. Indeed their function may be completely altered, as with rosemary tea which, when steeped for the correct time, is mildly soporiphic, but when left too long in the pot is quite the opposite.

If dried leaves are used 1 teaspoonful of herb for each cup and one for the pot is generally correct, although specific recipes will differ. Many of these dried herbs may now be bought in tea bags, but care must be taken that they are as fresh as possible. For teas made from *fresh* leaves, the proportion is three times as much as for dried. The fresh leaves should be torn, or slightly bruised by being squeezed in a cloth or tissue before putting in the pot. For teas made from seeds 1 tablespoon per 600ml (1 pint) is the dose.

Earthenware, china, porcelain, glass or enamel must be used for the pot or jug, never metal. The vessel should be warmed before the herbs are put in and the boiling water poured on. Generally speaking teas should steep for 5–10 minutes and then be strained into the cup. To increase the strength put in more leaves, do not increase the infusion time.

With the tea mixtures or tisanes, the herbalist wants to combine, strengthen, or slow down the effects of different medicinal plants, or to prevent disagreeable side effects. Plants yield their substances better when chopped up than when whole, and in these mixtures the proportions of the various constituents are balanced. Where nothing else is indicated the tea is to be drunk hot and unsweetened, or with the addition of honey or fruit juice, slowly in small sips, before or between meals. A tea cure should be taken consistently for three or four weeks.

The following three methods of preparation apply to all medicinal plants and tea mixtures. Other applications are specifically mentioned.

INFUSIONS: used for flowers or fine leaves.
Put 1–2 heaped teaspoonfuls or 2–3 pinches of herbs in a cup, pour boiling water over them, leave, covered, for 5–10 minutes to infuse, then strain.

DECOCTIONS: for coarser flowers and leaves, without stems.
Put 1–2 tablespoons of chopped herbs in a pan and pour half a litre of cold water over them. Bring to the boil and simmer lightly for 1–2 minutes covered, then leave to infuse for 10 minutes before straining into a thermos flask.

MACERATION: used for hard leaves, bark and roots.
Put 1–2 tablespoons of the chopped plant into half a litre of cold water and leave to soak for one hour. Bring to the boil, simmer over a very low heat for 10–15 minutes and then cover and leave to stand for 10 minutes. Strain into a thermos flask.

Headache tea

25g/0.9oz cowslip flowers
10g/0.35oz camomile flowers
5g/0.2oz arnica flowers
5g/0.2oz marigold petals
5g/0.2oz lavender
15g/0.5oz bergamot
5g/0.2oz peppermint leaves
25g/0.9oz blessed thistle
Make an infusion. For chronic headaches take half a cupful of tea every 2 hours. Put a cold compress of spirit of lavender on the forehead.

Nerve tea

10g/0.35oz lavender
15g/0.5oz orange blossom petals
10g/0.35oz lime flowers
10g/0.35oz rosemary leaves
5g/0.2oz bergamot petals
10g/0.35oz lemon balm leaves
20g/0.7oz hops
10g/0.35g woodruff
10g/0.35oz valerian root
Make an infusion. Take 1–2 cups an hour before going to bed. This can also be taken if necessary during the day.

Tea for the chest

15g/0.5oz coltsfoot
15g/0.5oz lime flowers
10g/0.35oz common mallow
10g/0.35oz holly
15g/0.5oz mallow
25g/0.9oz wild thyme
10g/0.35oz liquorice
Make a decoction. Sweeten with honey if necessary.

Tea for night sweats,

hot flushes during the menopause and for fits of faintness
40g/1.4oz sage leaves
10g/0.35oz rosemary
10g/0.35oz lemon balm
20g/0.7oz hops
10g/0.35oz hyssop
10g/0.35oz St John's wort
Make an infusion.

Tea for flu and colds

5g/0.2oz lavender
20g/0.7oz elderflower
25g/0.9oz meadowsweet
15g/0.5oz holly
15g/0.5oz dried oats
20g/0.7oz thyme
Make an infusion. Add two slices of lemon if necessary, and a coffeespoon of rum. Drink 1–2 cups, hot.

Tea for the circulation

5g/0.2oz lavender
15g/0.5oz cowslip
5g/0.2oz peppermint
5g/0.2oz rosemary
20g/0.7oz bayleaves
20g/0.7oz hawthorn
10g/0.35oz horsetail
20g/0.7oz mistletoe
Make a decoction. Take 2–4 cups daily for several weeks.

Tea for women's troubles

10g/0.35oz lady's mantle
10g/0.35oz silvermantle (or 20g/0.7oz lady's mantle)

15g/0.5oz St John's wort
5g/0.2oz dead nettle
15g/0.5oz silverweed
5g/0.2oz rosemary
10g/0.35oz lemon balm
10g/0.35oz camomile
10g/0.35oz yarrow
10g/0.35oz tormentil
Make a decoction. Also sit in a warm bath with a yarrow infusion added.

Tea to aid the digestion
10g/0.35oz centaury
10g/0.35oz nettle
5g/0.2oz wormwood
5g/0.2oz feverfew
20g/0.7oz camomile
10g/0.35oz lemon balm
10g/0.35oz elecampane
10g/0.35oz fennel
10g/0.35oz common mallow
10g/0.35oz yellow gentian
To cure indigestion, sip a third of a cup, slowly, every hour.

Tea to cure diarrhoea
15g/0.5oz silverweed
15g/0.5oz St John's wort
15g/0.5oz shepherd's purse
10g/0.35oz hyssop
10g/0.35oz caraway
20g/0.7oz bilberries
20g/0.7oz tormentil
Make a decoction. Take one cup every two hours.

Tea for arthritis
10g/0.35oz juniper berries
10g/0.35oz elderflower
10g/0.35oz goatsbeard
20g/0.7oz willow bark
20g/0.7oz birch leaves
15g/0.5oz restharrow
15g/0.5oz dwarf elder
Make a decoction. Take 3–4 cups daily. Avoid alcohol and nicotine.

A laxative tea
15g/0.5oz blackthorn flowers
15g/0.5oz elderflower
10g/0.35oz fennel seed
10g/0.35oz linseed
20g/0.7oz alder bark
10g/0.35oz dandelion root
10g/0.35oz rhubarb
10g/0.35oz senna
Drink one cup every evening, so that the bowels function the following morning.

Tea for liverishness
5g/0.2oz marigold
10g/0.35oz centaury
10g/0.35oz curled mint
10g/0.35oz feverfew
10g/0.35oz yarrow
20g/0.7oz boldo
5g/0.2oz wormwood
10g/0.35oz dandelion root
10g/0.35oz mouse-eared hawkweed
Make a decoction. Take a cup in the morning on an empty stomach and between meals. Avoid alcohol and nicotine.

Tea for the kidneys and bladder
5g/0.2oz marigold
10g/0.35oz bilberry
15g/0.5oz bearberry
10g/0.35oz nettle
10g/0.35oz horsetail
20g/0.7oz juniper
10g/0.35oz restharrow
A decoction. Take 4–5 half cups daily. Avoid alcohol and nicotine.

Tea against eczema
5g/0.2oz camomile
5g/0.2oz marigold
15g/0.5oz St John's wort
10g/0.35oz common mallow
25g/0.9oz herb robert
20g/0.7oz horsetail
20g/0.7oz sanicle
Use as compresses or to bathe skin.

Tea against sweaty feet

40g/1.4oz oak bark
20g/0.7oz horsetail
10g/0.35oz wild thyme
10g/0.35oz rosemary
20g/0.7oz tormentil

Make a maceration. Dilute a half litre with a litre of hot water. Bathe feet in this for 10 minutes, then rinse with cold water. Do not wear socks of synthetic fibre.

Tisanes

BERGAMOT a sleep-inducing nightcap. 1 teaspoon of bergamot per cup simmered for 10 minutes in an enamel or stainless steel pan, and sweetened with honey if liked. Alternatively bergamot may be made as a tea.

BILBERRY TEA Berries used must be carefully dried. Soak 1 tablespoon dried bilberries for some hours then drain and pour 2 pints boiling water over them, bring to the boil and remove from the heat. Allow to stand for 10 minutes then strain and serve hot. The *leaves* of bilberries, gathered in April and May may be made into a spring tea, particularly good for the overweight.

BLACKBERRY LEAVES are valuable if gathered in the spring as a tonic drink and the tea made with them is also good as a gargle.

CARAWAY SEEDS have a carminative or anti-flatulent effect and one cup after meals is suggested. Boiling water is poured over 1 teaspoon of bruised caraway seeds per cup, steeped for 10 minutes then strained.

CAMOMILE (*Mactricaria Chamomilla*) is a perfect digestive after-dinner tea. It has a soothing action on the digestive tract and upon the mucus membranes. An infusion is excellent for a mouthwash, for sore throats and following tooth extraction. It can also be used as a facial steam for a heavy cold or as an eyebath for sore eyelids. For both tea or lotion, take 1 teaspoon camomile flowers per cup in boiling water, steeped for no longer than 3–5 minutes.

ELDERFLOWER TEA A pleasant summer drink and also good for colds. Elderflowers mixed with lime flowers and camomile in equal parts also make an excellent tea in cases of flu or heavy colds. A teaspoon of dried elderflowers per cup plus one for the pot makes a sleep-inducing tea. An infusion of elderflowers and water is used for an eyebath and also has cosmetic properties if used as a skin lotion. A face pack may be made by adding elderflowers to yoghurt.

HORSETAIL TEA is astringent and antiseptic and also has cosmetic qualities, toning the skin and strengthening hair and nails. A teaspoon of the herb per cup should be soaked for several hours then boiled in the water for 10–15 minutes, and allowed to steep for another 10–15 minutes before straining.

JUNIPER BERRIES 1 teaspoon or 12–18 crushed berries are used per cup, boiling water is poured on and allowed to stand for 10 minutes. It can be sweetened with 1 teaspoon of honey if liked. This is often taken in cases of stomach or intestinal trouble. Juniper berries can also be used as a bath preparation.

LADY'S MANTLE TEA This is mainly used for female disorders, improving the functions of the female organs at puberty, throughout life, during pregnancy and particularly during the menopause. It is also astringent for the skin.

MARIGOLD PETAL TEA is soothing for intestinal conditions and also has cosmetic properties.

ROSEMARY TEA The fresh or dried leaves are used, young sprigs and flowering tops. This is a stimulant for the heart in the same way as rosemary wine. An infusion makes a splendid hair tonic.

SOLIDAGO TEA The upper part of the flowering plant should be dried. Boil the herb for 1 minute, allow to steep for 10 minutes then strain. 2–3 cups daily are taken in cases of inflammation of the bladder and kidneys.

VERBASCUM TEA is made from the yellow flowers, either fresh or dried. The flowers must be bright yellow. This is good for bronchial conditions; during an acute cold 2–3 cups a day may be taken, and it dramatically helps coughs.

YARROW TEA can be made from the leaves and flowers and is a digestive. The tea is effective also when made from dried yarrow. A teaspoon per cup with boiling water poured over.

COLTSFOOT TEA (Flowers collected March–May, leaves from May–July and dried carefully.) The tea has a cleansing and tonic effect because it is diuretic.

CENTAURY TEA improves the condition of liver and circulation of the blood. 1 teaspoon per cup. Steep in hot, not boiling, water and let it draw for 10 minutes. This is a good early morning drink, soothing and cleansing and good for the skin.

Other concoctions

ARNICA SCHNAPS
Place a handful of arnica blossoms in a wide necked glass, pour 300ml (0.5 pint) of fruit brandy over it and cover. Leave the glass to stand, sealed, for eight days in the sun. Filter it through a coffee filter into a bottle.

ROSEMARY WINE
Cut 5–6 fresh rosemary sprigs, chop finely with a kitchen knife, put them into a litre of white wine and let it stand for twenty days in a well sealed bottle. Filter it through a coffee filter and drink a little glass before meals.

ST JOHN'S OIL
Put a handful of open, or half open, St John's wort flower buds in a bowl, pour a little sun-flower oil on them and crush the flowers with a wooden spoon. Pour 300ml (0.5 pint) of sunflower oil on the mixture. Decant into a white bottle and place the mixture in the sun for 8–10 days. Then filter it through a clean linen cloth into a brown medicine bottle. This is used for burns, wounds and inflammation of the skin.

BIRCH HAIR LOTION
If birch trees are pruned or tapped in the spring they exude a lot of sap. This contains sugar and ferments very quickly. To 300ml (0.5 pint) of sap 1 decilitre of surgical spirit is added immediately. It is then scented with strong eau de cologne. This is used to massage into the scalp.

BATH FOR HELPING PERIOD PAINS
20g/0.7oz herb robert
20g/0.7oz golden rod
20g/0.7oz horsetail
10g/0.35oz mallow
20g/0.7oz oak bark
10g/0.35oz tormentil
Macerate all the ingredients to make a litre (1.75 pints) of concentrated tea. Put 200ml (6 fl oz) of the mixture into a bath of warm water, and bathe, morning and evening, for 15 minutes.

Herbs for Beauty

Herbs associated with the skin

Camomile flowers are soothing, cleansing and gently astringent

Coltsfoot leaves are soothing and prevent thread veins

Comfrey leaves and root are emollient and healing

Dandelion leaves and root are tonic and cleansing

Elder flowers are softening, soothing and cleansing

Horsetail non-fertile stems are astringent and strengthen nails and close pores

Ladys Mantle leaves are healing and astringent

Lime flowers are soothing, cleansing and bleaching

Marigold leaves and flowers are healing and soothing

Mint leaves are healing, stimulating, antiseptic

Plantain leaves are astringent and cleansing

Rosemary leaves are invigorating and astringent

Sage leaves are deodorant, astringent, close pores and revitalise tissue

Nettle leaves, seeds, and roots are cleansing, toning, and improve circulation

Thyme leaves are deodorant and antiseptic

Yarrow leaves and flowers are strongly astringent

Herbal Foot Bath

A large handful of fresh or 3 tbsps dried herbs . . . sage, thyme, lavender, marjoram or bay

1 tbsp sea salt

Put the herbs and salt in a large bowl with boiling water, allow to cool and use as a foot-bath for tired feet. This has a marked refreshing and restorative effect on the whole body.

Elderflower Milk Bath

300ml/0.5 pint milk

100g/4oz fresh or 50g/2oz dried elderflowers

Infuse the flowers in the milk for one to four hours. This in a bath will soften the skin, it can also be made with camomile or lime flowers.

Simple Lotion

A handful of fresh camomile, meadow-sweet, elder or lime flowers

75ml/3 fl oz warm milk, cream, butter-milk or whey

honey

Soak the flowers in the liquid in a covered pan for three hours. Strain, reheat, and dissolve a little honey in the liquid. A spoonful of oatmeal, bran, or wheat germ will thicken the lotion. Keep refrigerated and use within a week.

Camomile and Cucumber Lotion

75ml/3 fl oz camomile infusion

350g/12oz cucumber

6 teasps glycerine

Chop the cucumber finely and squeeze out all the juice. Slightly warm the infusion and stir in the glycerine, and then the cucumber juice. Cool and bottle. Refrigerate. A softening lotion.

Elderflower Cream

2 level tbsps dried elderflowers or enough
fresh flowers to be just covered by
the oil
150ml/¼ pint almond or other oil
4 teasps lanolin
1 teasp honey

Warm the oil and lanolin in the top
of a double boiler. Add the flowers
and simmer for 30 minutes. Cool, pot
up and label. An emollient cream.

Marigold Cream

75ml/3 fl oz strong marigold infusion
6 teasps melted beeswax
6 teasps lanolin
¼ teasp borax
6 tbsps almond or other oil

Warm the wax, lanolin and oil in the
top of a double saucepan. Warm the
infusion in a separate saucepan and
dissolve the borax thoroughly in the
solution. Take both pans from the
heat and combine the contents
gradually, then beat up or whisk
together until cooled and thickened.
Stir in 2 capsules of wheatgerm oil
for extra vitamin E. Pot and label.

Comfrey Cream Cleaner

150ml/¼ pint infusion comfrey leaves
150ml/¼ pint almond or other oil
1 teasp borax
2 tbsps melted beeswax
2 tbsps cocoa butter
2 teasps honey

Melt the oil, beeswax and cocoa butter
in a double saucepan. Warm the
infusion in another pan. Stir in the
borax and honey and dissolve.
Remove both pans from the stove,
amalgamate the mixtures and beat
with a wooden spoon or electric
mixer. The cream will thicken as it
cools. Pot and label.

Herbs for the hair

Camomile encourages hair growth

and sooths scalp irritation
Horsetail strengthens the hair
Lime flowers soften and cleanse hair
Marigold petals lighten hair colour
Mullein flowers lighten hair colour
Rosemary the best all round hair tonic
and conditioner, leaves and
flowering tops give lustre and body
and slightly darken the hair
Sage leaves are tonic and conditioning
and slightly darken the hair
Soapwort leaves and roots cleanse
Nettle leaves help prevent dandruff,
and are tonic and conditioning

Rosemary Oil Conditioner

2 drops oil of rosemary
1 tbsp glycerine
1 egg (yolk only for dry hair)
1 tbsp almond oil
1 tbsp lanolin

Combine the oils, glycerine and lanolin
in the top of a double saucepan and
warm gently. Remove from the heat
and beat in the egg. A conditioner
that can be rubbed into the scalp after
shampooing. Leave on for 10 minutes
and rinse well.

Soapwort Shampoo

1 tbsp grated or powdered soapwort root
A handful of fresh or 1 tbsp dried
camomile flowers, or other herbs
300ml/½ pint boiling water

Pour the boiling water on to the
soapwort and camomile, cover and
leave to infuse until cool. The
camomile adds additional strength
and scent to the shampoo.

A mild shampoo

2 tbsps of a strong infusion of herbs
1 tbsp pure baby shampoo or of dissolved
unscented soap

Use an infusion of sage for dark hair,
yarrow for oily hair, marigold petals
for fair hair, a mixture of nettle and
burdock for dandruff.

Bibliography

The Concise British Flora in Colour, W. Keble Martin, Ebury Press and Michael Joseph, 1974.

The Oxford Book of Wild Flowers, Ary and Gregory, Oxford University Press, 1960.

The Herb and Spice Book, Sarah Garland, Frances Lincoln Publishers Ltd, 1979.

Herbs for Health and Cookery, Lowenfeld and Back, Pan, 1971.

A Guide to Medicinal Plants, Schauenberg and Paris, Lutterworth Press, 1977.

A Modern Herbal, Mrs M. Grieve, Penguin Books, 1976.

Health Secrets of Plants and Herbs, Maurice Mességué, William Collins, 1979.

Sources of further information

The British Homoeopathic Association, 27a Devonshire Street, London W1N 1RJ.

The Herb Society, 34 Boscobel Place, London SW1W 9PE.

Index